KU-496-454

THE HEALTHY DIET CALORIE COUNTER

dbp

DUNCAN BAIRD PUBLISHERS
LONDON

REFERENCES

J. S. Bainbridge, *Diet for the Million* (Williams & Norgate Ltd, UK, 1926); R. Ballentine, *Diet & Nutrition – A Holistic Approach* (The Himalayan International Institute, US, 1982); H. G. Bieler, *Food Is Your Best Medicine* (Neville Spearman, UK, 1968); M. Bircher-Benner, *Food Science for All* (The C. W. Daniel Company, UK, 1939); W. Chan, J. Brown & D. H. Buss, *Miscellaneous Foods,* supplement to *McCance & Widdowson's The Composition of Foods* (Royal Society of Chemistry & MAFF, UK, 1994); H. Crawley, *Food Portion Sizes* (MAFF & HMSO, UK, 1992); S. Davies & A. Stewart, *Nutritional Medicine* (Pan Books, UK, 1987); Food Standards Agency, *McCance & Widdowson's The Composition of Foods,* 6th summary edition (Royal Society of Chemistry, UK, 2002); J. S. Garrow, W. P. T. James & A. Ralph, *Human Nutrition & Dietetics,* 10th edition (Churchill Livingstone, UK, 2000); B. Holland, et al, *Cereals & Cereal Products,* supplement to *McCance & Widdowson's The Composition of Foods* (Royal Society of Chemistry & MAFF, UK, 1988); B. Holland et al, *Fruits & Nuts,* supplement to *McCance & Widdowson's The Composition of Foods* (Royal Society of Chemistry & MAFF, UK, 1992); B. Holland et al, *Vegetables, Herbs & Spices,* supplement to *McCance & Widdowson's The Composition of Foods* (Royal Society of Chemistry & MAFF, UK, 1991); B. Holland et al, *Vegetable Dishes,* supplement to *McCance & Widdowson's The Composition of Foods* (Royal Society of Chemistry & MAFF, UK, 1992); R. E. Kowalski, *The 8-Week Cholesterol Cure* (Thorson, UK, 1990); J. G. G. Ledingham & D. A. Warrell (eds), *Concise Oxford Textbook of Medicine* (Oxford University Press, UK, 2000); T. Lobstein, *Fast Food Facts* (The London Food Commision, Camden Press, UK, 1988); The London Food Commission, *Food Adulteration and How to Beat It* (Unwin Hyman Ltd, UK, 1988); R. Mackarness, *Eat Fat and Grow Slim* (Fontana, UK, 1980); L. Mervyn, *The Dictionary of Minerals* (Thorsons, UK, 1985); L. Mervyn, *The Dictionary of Vitamins* (Thorsons, UK, 1984); J. L. Mount, *The Food and Health of Western Man* (Precision Press, UK, 1979); M. Murray & J. Pizzorno, *An Encyclopaedia of Natural Medicine* (Macdonald Optima, US, 1990); Parents for Safe Food, *Safe Food Handbook* (Ebury Press, 1990); A. A. Paul et al, *Amino Acids & Fatty Acids,* supplement to *McCance & Widdowson's The Composition of Foods* (Royal Society of Chemistry & MAFF, UK, 1992); W. A. Price, *Nutrition and Physical Degeneration* (The Price-Pottenger Nutrition Foundation, 1982); N. Rowley, *Basic Clinical Science* (Hodder & Stoughton, UK, 1994); J. Salmon, *Dietary Reference Values – A Guide* (Department of Health & HMSO, UK, 1991); S. Stender, J. Dyerberg, G. Hølmer, L. Ovesen & B. Sandstrøm, *Transfedtsyrernes Betydning for Sundheden* (Ernæringsrådet, Denmark, 1995); Weight Watchers, *1, 2, 3 Success* (Weight Watchers Ltd, UK, 1996); Weight Watchers, *Selection Guide – The A–Z of Selection Values* (Weight Watchers International Inc., UK, 1993); M. R. Werbach, *Nutritional Influences on Illness* (Thorsons, UK, 1989); World Cancer Research Fund in association with American Institute of Cancer Research, *Food Nutrition and the Prevention of Cancer – A Global Perspective* (American Institute for Cancer Research, USA, 1997); manufacturer and on-line data.

THE HEALTHY DIET CALORIE COUNTER Kirsten Hartvig

To Nic

Conceived, created and designed by
Duncan Baird Publishers Ltd
Sixth Floor, Castle House
75–76 Wells Street
London W1T 3QH

Copyright © Duncan Baird Publishers 2004
Text copyright © Kirsten Hartvig 2004
Copyright of photographs © Duncan Baird Publishers 2004

The right of Kirsten Hartvig to be identified as the Author of this text has been asserted in accordance with the Copyright, Designs and Patents Act of 1988.

All rights reserved. No part of this publication may be reproduced or utilized in any form or by any means electronic or mechanical, including photocopying, recording, or by any information storage and retrieval system now known or hereafter invented, without the prior written permission of the Publisher.

Managing Editor: Julia Charles
Editors: Lucy Latchmore & James Hodgson
Managing Designer: Dan Sturges
Designer: Adelle Morris
Commissioned Photography: Matthew Ward

A Cataloguing-in-Publication record for this book is available from the British Library.

ISBN: 1-84483-015-2

10 9 8 7 6 5 4 3

Typeset in Frutiger
Colour reproduction by Scanhouse, Malaysia
Printed and bound in China by Imago

Publisher's Note: The information in this book is intended only as a guide to following a healthy diet and is not meant as a substitute for medical advice and treatment. People with special dietary requirements of any kind should consult appropriate medical professionals before changing their diet. The tables have been compiled using data derived from a variety of sources including manufacturer data. The literature sources are listed together with other references on page 4 (see opposite). Some values have been estimated based on similar foods.

ACKNOWLEDGMENTS
The author would like to thank Judy Barratt, Geoffrey Cannon, Julia Charles, Peter Firebrace, Peter Goldman, James Hodgson, Lucy Latchmore, Jennifer Maughan, Françoise Nassivet, Amanda Preston, Nic Rowley, Bob Saxton, Joyce Thomas, Linda Wilkinson, as well as all those friends, colleagues, teachers, students and clients who, knowingly or unknowingly, have contributed to this book.

Contents

Introduction 8

Part 1: Calories 10

All about calories 12

How many calories do we need? 24

Part 2: Carbohydrates, Fats & Proteins 30

All about carbohydrates 32

All about proteins 38

All about fats 42

Carbohydrate, fat and protein tables 49

Fruit 50

Nuts and seeds 54

Vegetables and pulses 56

Vegetable dishes 60

Meat and meat dishes 64

Fish and fish dishes 68

Dairy products 70

Fats and oils 74

Grains, cereals, breads 76

Biscuits, cakes, puddings 80

Sugar products 84

Soups and sauces 86

Pickles and savouries 88

Drinks 90

Part 3: Vitamins, Minerals & Trace Elements 94

All about vitamins 96

Vitamin tables 119

Fruit 120

Nuts and seeds 124

Vegetables and pulses 126

Vegetable dishes 130

Meat and meat dishes 134

Fish and fish dishes 138
Dairy products 140
Fats and oils 144
Grains, cereals, breads 146
Biscuits, cakes, puddings 150
Sugar products 154
Soups and sauces 156
Pickles and savouries 158
Drinks 160
All about minerals 164
All about trace elements 172
Mineral and trace element tables 179
Fruit 180
Nuts and seeds 184
Vegetables and pulses 186
Vegetable dishes 190
Meat and meat dishes 194
Fish and fish dishes 198
Dairy products 200
Fats and oils 204
Grains, cereals, breads 206
Biscuits, cakes, puddings 210
Sugars products 214
Soups and sauces 216
Pickles and savouries 218
Drinks 220

Part 4: Diets 224

Diets and dieting 226
Diet plans 236

Index 240

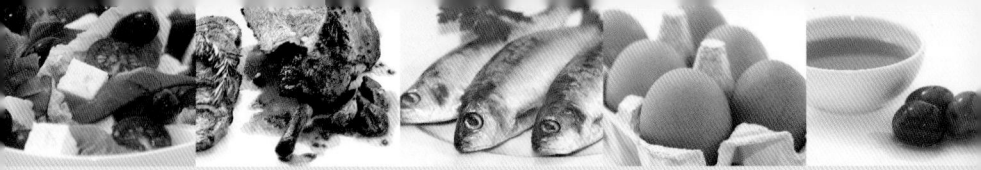

INTRODUCTION

Obesity is now a major threat to health. A staggering 61 per cent of American adults are overweight and obesity among children is increasing at an alarming rate. In most cases, the cause is simple – eating too many empty calories.

Empty calories are those that provide energy but little else of nutritional value. A chocolate bar, for example, may contain the same number of calories as an avocado, but it is not nearly as nutritious. If our food consists mainly of empty calories, we become both overweight and undernourished. The lack of vital nutrients in an empty-calorie diet lowers our resistance to disease and saps our stamina, making it difficult for the body to function properly.

This book is about quality calories – calories that come from foods that make you healthy. Whether you are trying to lose weight, or simply want to maintain your current weight in the healthiest possible way, meeting your daily calorie needs with quality calories automatically provides your body with all the

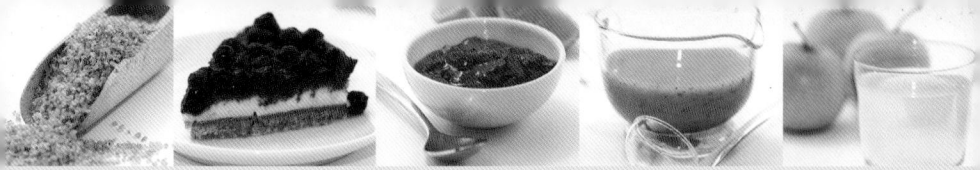

essential nutrients that it needs for good health. Quality calories are satisfying and nourishing, and make it easy to avoid over-eating. The more quality calories your diet contains, the less space there will be for empty calories.

High-protein diets and calorie counting can produce short-term weight reduction but sustainable weight loss involves improving the quality of each calorie you eat. High-protein diets work because the hunger centre in the brain is sensitive to protein intake. However, the body uses protein primarily to create body structures, and only converts it into energy as a last resort. While a high-protein diet may be nourishing, protein overload can also cause health problems, and it is important for long-term health to eat foods that are well-balanced nutritionally. This does not mean boring meals and endless restrictions, it means enjoying more of the huge variety of inexpensive, widely available, energy-giving foods that are good for your body and good for you – foods rich in quality calories.

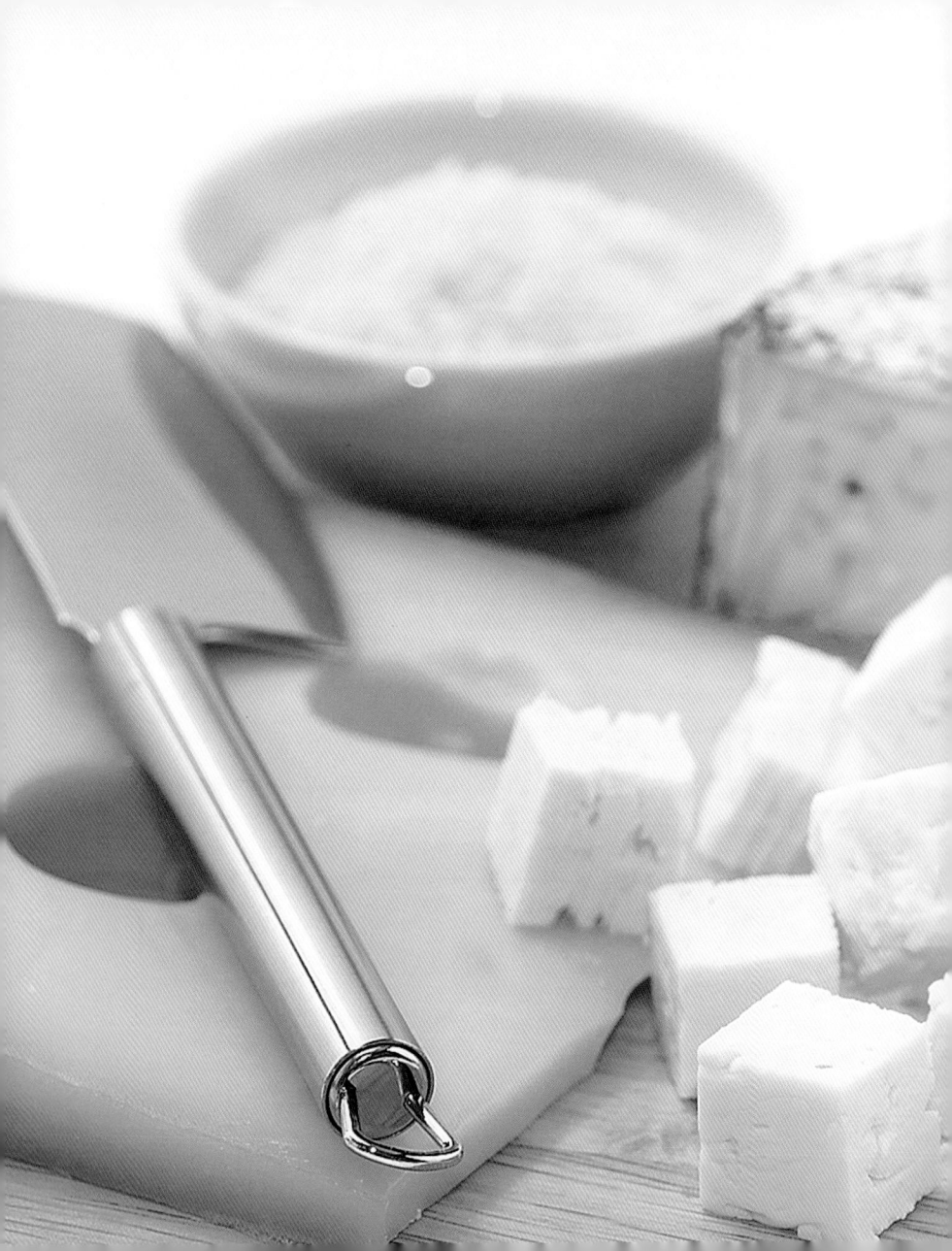

Part 1
CALORIES

Part 1 lays the foundation for the rest of this book. We start by exploring the background to calorie counting. We learn about the complex relationship between calories, food and dieting, the role of appetite in regulating calorie intake, and how this mechanism can go wrong when we eat empty calories rather than quality calories. Next we are introduced to the nutrient tables. We discover the unique quality-calorie points system and the Quality Calorie Targets, and are guided through the process of using these tools to improve the nutritional quality of our diet. This is followed by a discussion of obesity and eating disorders. The section concludes with an explanation of the factors affecting our energy needs, and a step-by-step procedure for calculating our optimum calorie intake.

All about calories

CALORIES AND ENERGY

A calorie is a unit of heat energy, technically defined as "the energy needed to raise the temperature of one gram of water by one degree centigrade". In the body, the process of metabolism converts the calories contained in food into the energy we need to live. As even small amounts of food can contain thousands of calories of energy, it has become standard practice to express food energy in terms of kilocalories (where 1 kilocalorie = 1000 calories). One gram of carbohydrate provides just under four kilocalories of energy, one gram of protein provides four kilocalories, and fat provides nine kilocalories per gram. Fat is more "calorie-dense" than protein or carbohydrate because it is designed for the compact storage of energy.

It is possible, using charts and tables, to work out exactly how many calories we need for our age, height and activity level. However, the bottom line is simple: we need as many as we use. Children use calories for growth and are usually very active; but they are also small so they need fewer calories than adults overall. Older people are generally less active, so they

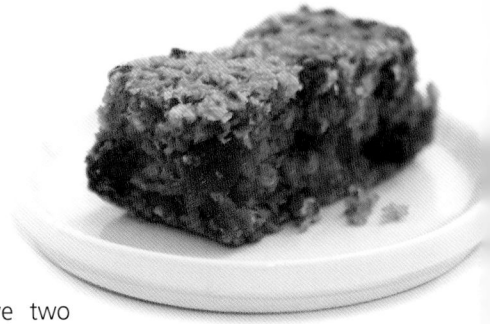

also need fewer calories. Pregnant and nursing mothers need more calories than average women because they have two mouths to feed. Overweight bodies use up more energy than non-overweight bodies, because they carry around extra weight.

If we eat more calories than we need, the extra energy released from food is converted into fat and stored for later use. If we don't use up our fat stores, we become overweight.

CALORIES AND APPETITE

The appetite is our natural in-built calorie counter that ensures we take in enough energy to fuel our daily activities. It makes us feel hungry when we need energy, and full when we've eaten enough. If we eat healthy food, the appetite does the calorie counting automatically. So, to take a major step toward maintaining a healthy weight, all we need to do is learn to pay attention to the signals that our bodies give us about what we need, rather than to what our eyes tell us we want.

EMPTY CALORIES VERSUS QUALITY CALORIES

For most of us, empty calories form a substantial part of our daily diet, making it hard for us to hear the quiet voice of healthy appetite (see box, opposite). Processed foods that combine carbohydrates with fats (cream cakes, for example) often produce feelings of immediate satisfaction when they are eaten. However, these feelings don't last because the calories are not accompanied by other nutrients that the body needs. As a result we are tempted to eat more empty calories and risk being trapped in a vicious circle of poor nutrition and increasing weight. More people pig out on chocolate biscuits than on carrots, but even if you were to binge on carrots, the damage in terms of calories would be minimal: four chocolate biscuits contain over 500 kilocalories, while four carrots contain just 35 kilocalories. Whether you are interested in slimming, or simply want to maintain a healthy weight, the vital step is to make the change from a calorie-dense, nutrient-deficient empty-calorie diet to a nutrient-rich, quality-calorie diet (see box, p.16).

Using the tables in Part 2 and Part 3, you will be able to identify foods with a high quality-calorie count (that is, foods

A typical empty-calorie diet

Breakfast	White buttered toast with jam, coffee with milk and sugar
Morning snack	Chocolate bar, cup of coffee with milk and sugar
Lunch	Hamburger in a white bun with fries, a soda
Afternoon snack	Tea with milk and sugar, cake or biscuits
Dinner	A few drinks followed by a processed food meal, with perhaps another few drinks

Although this diet provides plenty of calories, it is high in saturated fat, protein and refined carbohydrate, and contains little useful nourishment. Excess saturated fat leads to the formation of dangerous fatty deposits in the blood vessels; excess protein causes bad breath and kidney problems; excess refined carbohydrates disrupt energy levels by upsetting blood-sugar balance; and calories derived from alcohol place strain on the liver.

with a high ratio of nutrients to calories). Eating more of these foods will improve the nutritional quality of your diet, and make it easier to keep up your energy levels with fewer calories overall. Simply by eating more quality calories, you will become healthier and find it easier to maintain an optimum weight in the long term.

In addition, you can use the information on vitamins, minerals and trace elements contained in Part 3 to help you

Benefits of quality calories

Quality-calorie counting will help you to create a diet that is:

- high in fibre and complex carbohydrates
- high in polyunsaturates and essential fatty acids
- a rich and balanced source of protein and essential amino acids
- rich in all important minerals and trace elements
- high in natural antioxidants
- low in fat
- low in cholesterol
- low in saturated fats
- low in hydrogenated fats and trans fats
- low in refined sugar
- free from harmful artificial additives

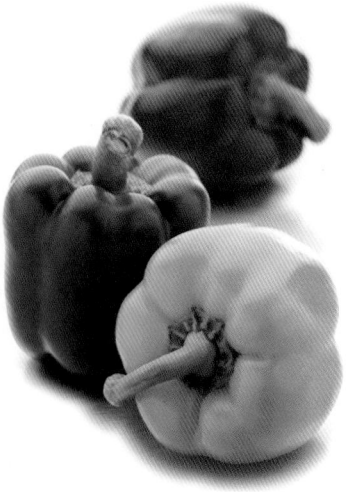

monitor your intake of essential micronutrients, and to learn about their importance in the maintenance of health and the treatment of disease. The descriptions of each vitamin and mineral enable you to check whether you may be suffering from a deficiency, and you can then use the tables to increase your intake of particular micronutrients by modifying your diet instead of taking expensive supplements.

QUALITY-CALORIE COUNTING

The tables in Parts 2 and 3 have two special features to help you optimize the nutritional quality of your diet. First, calorie counts for different foods are listed "per average portion", which means you don't have to weigh or measure anything to work out your calorie intake. Second, each food is rated according to a unique quality-calorie points system, devised so that the most nutritious foods (those that are low in saturated fat, contain the right amount of protein, the right kind of sugar, and plenty of vitamins and minerals) receive the highest scores. Foods that score fewer than 50 points are the most unbalanced. This does not mean they have no nutritional value, but that the balance of nutrients they contain is far from ideal.

The proteins, carbohydrates, fats, fibre, vitamins, minerals, trace elements and phytochemicals contained within the calories we eat give us energy to perform our daily tasks, and also help to prevent illness and promote healing. If you cut down on calories to lose weight, it is crucial that the food you eat has the right balance of nutrients. Choosing low-calorie foods with a high quality-calorie score ensures that your dietary needs are met while you are losing weight.

Follow these steps when using the Quality Calorie Guide to optimize your diet:

1 Use the calorie-intake tables on p.29 to work out how many calories you need each day based on your height, weight, sex, age and activity level. Note down the figure.

2 Carry a notebook and pen with you everywhere for the next seven days. Each time you eat something, write it down. You don't have to weigh or measure anything, just make a note of how many portions you eat of which foods.

3 At the end of each day, use the tables to work out the total number of calories you have consumed that day by adding together the "kcals per portion" for each portion of food you have eaten. Note down the figure.

4 Next, add together the quality-calorie points for each portion of food you have eaten during the day. Divide this total by the number of portions you have eaten. This gives you your average quality-calorie score for the day. Note the figure.

5 At the end of the week, add all seven daily calorie-intake figures together, and divide the total by seven to find your average daily calorie intake. Compare this figure with your optimum calorie intake. If your average daily intake is more than 200 calories higher than the ideal, you risk gaining weight. If it is more than 200 calories below the ideal, your weight will tend to diminish over time.

6 Look back at your average quality-calorie scores for each day. The higher the daily score, the better the nutritional quality of your diet. A daily score of 50 or less suggests that your diet contains too many empty calories.

7 Use the results of your analysis together with the tables in Part 2 and Part 3 to optimize your calorie intake and increase your quality-calorie scores.

QUALITY CALORIE TARGETS

The tables also provide you with a "Quality Calorie Target" (QCT) for the nutrients contained in different foods. This is worked out in accordance with the WHO recommended daily amounts and shows, at a glance, how close the nutrient content of a portion of any particular food is to the ideal. For proteins, carbohydrates and fats, the QCTs indicate the ideal percentages of calories that should be derived from each of the three nutrients. You can compare these figures with the percentages given for particular foods to ensure that your diet provides a balanced source of calories.

For vitamins, minerals, trace elements, fibre and essential fatty acids, the tables give the amount of each nutrient per portion of food in milligrams (mg) or micrograms (µg). By comparing these figures with the QCTs, you can work out how many portions you need to eat of particular foods to meet your daily requirements for each nutrient. (The body has a great capacity to store most nutrients, so you don't need to meet the target for every nutrient every day.) For example, suppose you wanted to optimize your zinc intake. Look at your diet record for day 1. Using the tables in Part 3, note the zinc content of each portion of food eaten during the day. Add the figures together. If the total is less than the zinc QCT of 9.4 mg, you are not eating enough zinc. Repeat the exercise for days 2–7. If you find your zinc intake is consistently low, use the tables to find foods that are high in zinc, and include more of these in your diet.

OBESITY AND EATING DISORDERS

Obesity means excess body fat, and is usually caused by a mixture of poor eating habits, lack of health education, metabolic disorders, depression, genetic predisposition and various social factors. It is also associated with a number of serious medical conditions, including coronary heart disease and cancer. One in six American children are overweight, and it is estimated that the obesity epidemic will cost Americans $260 billion a year in treatment by 2010.

People who are overweight clearly eat more calories than they use, and may have an altered sensitivity to hunger and fullness. This may be linked to reduced psychological resistance to sensory stimuli such as sight, smell and taste. Watching television is strongly associated with obesity because it provides strong sensory stimuli while promoting a sedentary lifestyle and lowering metabolic rate. This combination induces a trance-like state that makes it difficult to get up from the sofa and do something active.

To complicate matters, fat cells seem to have been designed to make dieting difficult. If, as a result of calorie restriction, fat cells become smaller, they send increasingly powerful signals to the brain asking to be fed, resulting in an overpowering urge to eat. The larger the number of fat cells, the stronger the urge, which explains why when fat people (who have more fat cells) follow severe diets (which shrink their fat cells rapidly), they frequently suffer a "rebound" effect from dieting and put on more weight after the diet than they lost by following it. In fact, studies suggest that only five per cent of obese people are able to slim down to and maintain an "ideal" body weight in the long term, which explains the continued proliferation of books on diet and dieting. (A wise physician once said that the more treatments

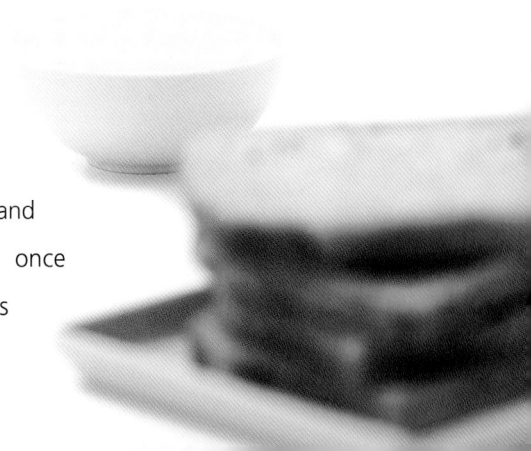

that are available for a disease, the less likely it is that any of them actually work.)

Maximizing sustainable weight loss involves losing weight slowly (between 0.5 and 1 lb a week). If you want to lose a pound a week, you must use up 500 calories more than you eat each day, which can be achieved by taking half an hour of aerobic exercise daily. A regular meal pattern (with little or no snacking) makes it easier to refrain from binge eating, and food containing plenty of fibre helps to keep the digestive system occupied. Also ensure that every calorie you eat is of the high nutritional quality to help your body resist cravings.

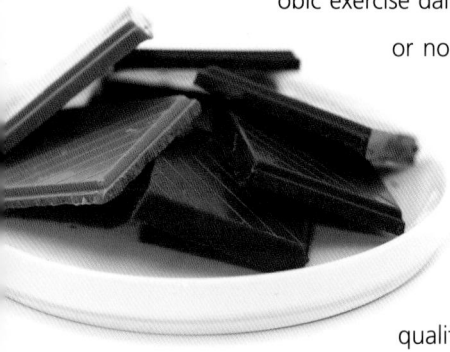

Recent research suggests that up to 30 per cent of obese people suffer from binge eating, a condition associated with eating disorders such as anorexia and bulimia nervosa. Binge eaters are more likely to be depressed and have anxiety disorders, such as panic attacks and post traumatic stress problems.

Both anorexics and bulimics have a distorted attitude to food. They suffer feelings of unworthiness and of being controlled, which are often rooted in rigid family patterns that can be hard to treat. Anorexia is characterized by persistent, active refusal of food, leading to profound weight loss. It is most common in young women, and leads to irregular or absent periods, strange eating habits, a disturbed body image and sometimes depression. If untreated it can prove fatal.

Bulimia is closely related to anorexia, and bulimics are similarly obsessed with body weight and size. They use vomiting, laxatives, diuretics, dieting, fasting or strenuous exercise to lose weight while at the same time indulging in repeated and uncontrollable bingeing.

All cases of binge eating, whether associated with obesity or eating disorders, should be treated medically, but there are simple self-help strategies which can alleviate some of the difficulties. Avoiding refined sugar, junk food, caffeine, alcohol and recreational drugs helps to stabilize blood-sugar levels, improve metabolism and bring greater inner clarity. Eating regular meals containing foods high in calcium, magnesium, zinc, B-vitamins and vitamin C also helps in this. Getting enough sleep, allowing time for creative expression and spending time outdoors assists in removing internal clutter.

How many calories do we need?

ENERGY NEEDS

A living body is rather like an internal combustion engine, burning fuel and oxygen to release energy, and giving off carbon dioxide and other waste products. This energy is used to maintain healthy functioning of the body and support activity. Not all the energy contained in food is available to the body. This is for two reasons: first, not all the food we eat is absorbed through the digestive tract (99 per cent of carbohydrate, 95 per cent of fat, and 92 per cent of protein is absorbed in fact); second, not all the protein we absorb is converted into energy – some of it is incorporated into the structure of body tissues.

Of the energy that is available, a great deal is used to maintain the basal metabolic rate (BMR). This is a measure of the energy needed to fuel all basic life functions while we are at rest. As well as the BMR, physical activity accounts for about 20 to 40 per cent of our energy use, with digestion, temperature regulation and coping with the after-effects of physical exertion accounting for the rest.

There are a number of factors that cause variations in energy needs between individuals:

- **Body size** – The bigger you are, the more energy you will need to perform the same activities. Energy use is also affected by body composition. A well-muscled body burns more energy than a fat body (which explains why it is easier to keep a fit body in trim).
- **Age** – Babies use a lot of energy to keep warm, and children and teenagers need extra energy to grow and fuel their often vigorous physical activities. As we get older, our metabolism slows down, our body tissues become more fatty, and we tend to become less active. Consequently, we need a lower intake of energy to maintain a healthy weight.
- **Sex** – Men generally need more calories than women because their body tissues contain less fat, their BMR is higher, and they are (on average) bigger. Pregnant women need extra energy to support the growth of the baby, and breastfeeding mothers require extra energy for producing milk.

- **Diet** – Overeating increases the BMR by five to ten per cent, while dieting reduces it by the same amount. Herein lies the paradox of weight loss: if you eat less to try to lose weight, your BMR drops, which means that your capacity to burn calories also diminishes. In effect, this means that dieting without an increase in physical activity is unlikely to produce sustainable weight loss. Aerobic exercise helps the process of weight reduction in three ways. First, it draws on energy stores while you are doing it, as well as during the following day when your body is recovering and readjusting. Second, exercise encourages the development of muscle, which raises the BMR. This means that you burn more calories at rest as well as when exercising. Third, exercise improves the circulation, enhances the absorption, digestion and metabolism of food, and helps the body to rid itself of waste products.
- **Activity** – It is normal to eat more if you use a lot of energy for physical activity: athletes and heavy-manual workers have increased energy needs to match their energy output.
- **Climate** – Keeping the right body temperature consumes energy – shivering to keep warm and sweating to keep cool both use up extra calories.

- **Genetic factors** – These account for variations in BMR of up to ten per cent in people of the same age, sex and body weight.
- **Hormonal state** – Thyroid over-activity increases energy expenditure, while thyroid under-activity reduces it. In women, the BMR is higher after ovulation. During pregnancy, the BMR falls initially, then increases as body weight increases.
- **Psychological state** – Anxiety and chronic stress increase energy expenditure.
- **Drugs** – Stimulants, such as nicotine and caffeine, increase energy expenditure. Amphetamines and other stimulants are sometimes used in treatment of obesity for this reason. Beta-blockers (often used in the treatment of hypertension and heart disease) decrease energy expenditure and can cause weight gain.
- **Disease** – Fevers, tumours and the physiological problems caused by severe burns all increase the BMR.

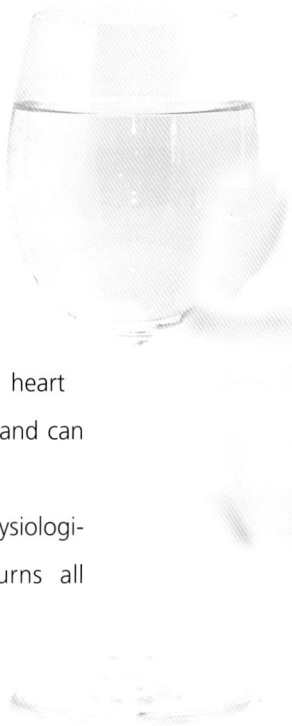

BODY MASS INDEX (BMI)

The Body Mass Index (BMI) provides a simple method of checking whether your weight is right for your height and build.

1. Write down your weight in kilograms (for example, 70).
2. Measure your height in metres (for example, 1.7).
3. Multiply this number by itself (for example, if you are 1.7 m tall, you would multiply 1.7 x 1.7 = 2.89).
4. Divide your weight by your height multiplied by itself (in this example, 70 / 2.89 = 24.22). This figure is your BMI.

Though simple to calculate, the BMI provides a powerful way of correlating weight to the likelihood of illness. Individuals with a high BMI are more likely to suffer from diabetes, hypertension and cardiovascular disease, as well as depression, respiratory disease and ulcers.

The body mass index is interpreted as follows:

BMI		BMI	
under 20	= underweight	30–35	= obese
20–25	= healthy weight	over 35	= seriously obese
25–30	= overweight		

Optimium calorie-intake tables grouped according to age and sex

Children and young people (aged 1-18)

Average daily energy need (moderate activity)

AGE	BOYS	GIRLS
1–3 years	1250 kcal	1175 kcal
4–6 years	1700 kcal	1550 kcal
7–10 years	1975 kcal	1750 kcal
11–14 years	2225 kcal	1850 kcal
15–18 years	2750 kcal	2100 kcal

Adults

Average daily energy need (moderate activity)

AGE	MEN	WOMEN
19–59 years	2700 kcal	2050 kcal
60–75 years	2350 kcal	1900 kcal
75+ years	2100 kcal	1800 kcal

ADJUSTMENTS

- When involved in heavy activity or vigorous exercise add 500 kcal per day.
- If leading a sedentary lifestyle subtract 150 kcal per day.
- During pregnancy add 200 kcal per day during the last 3 months.
- While breastfeeding add 500 to 600 kcal per day during the first 6 months. After that add between 250 and 550 depending on how much of the baby's energy and nutrient needs are supplied by breastfeeding. As soon as weaning begins, the mother's energy needs begin to fall to pre-pregnancy levels.

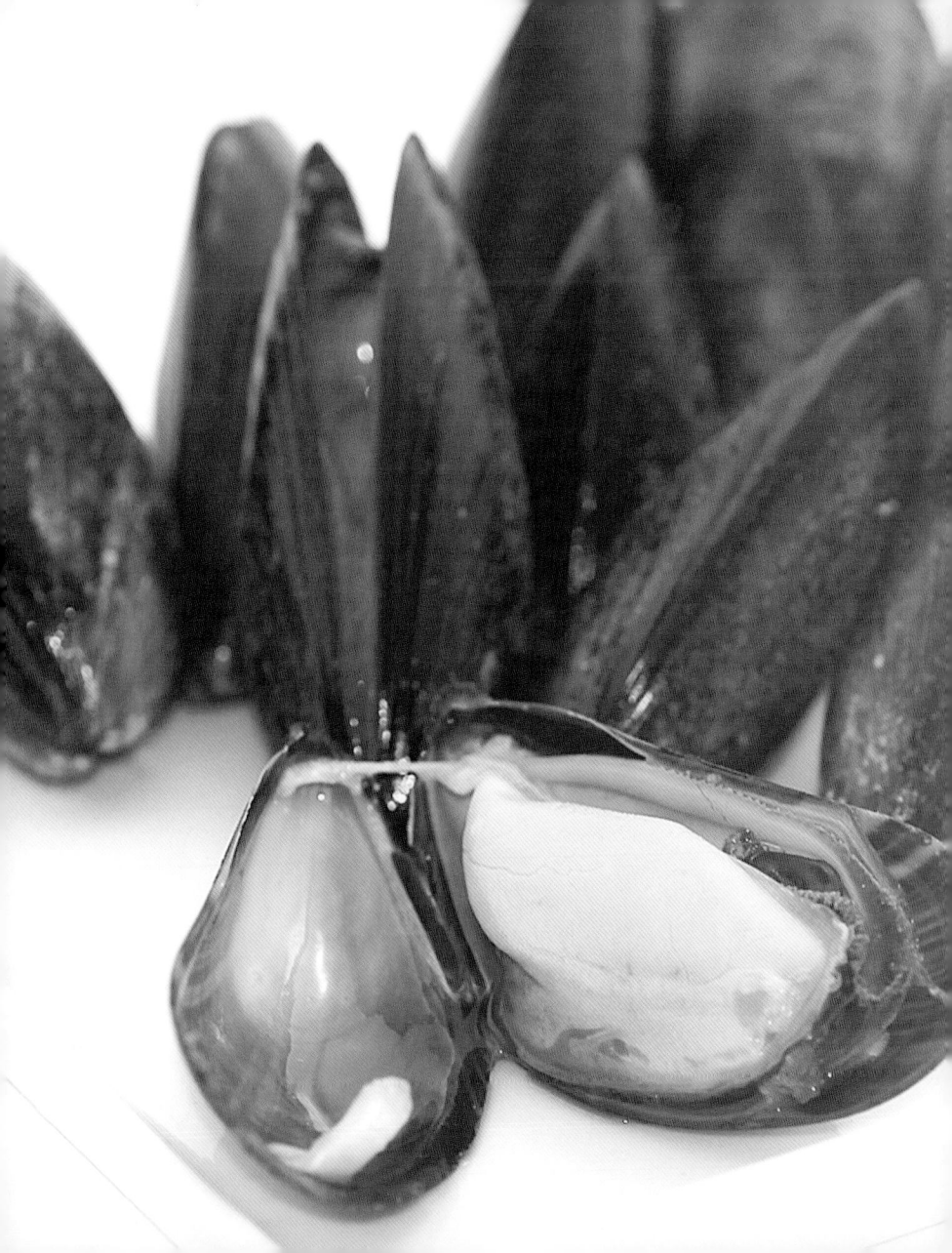

Part 2
CARBOHYDRATES, FATS & PROTEINS

In this part we discover essential nutritional facts about carbohydrates, proteins and fats in food. Working through each in turn, we learn of their structure, their function within the body and the relative proportions that we need of each for optimum health. We explore the differences between sugars and starches, plant and animal proteins and the various types of fat, finding out which forms are the most beneficial to health. This is supplemented with dietary tips for meeting our daily requirements for fibre, essential amino acids and essential fatty acids.

This information is followed by nutritional tables, which detail the calorie, protein, carbohydrate and fat content of a range of foods, enabling you to create a more balanced diet.

All about carbohydrates

There are many types of carbohydrates, and most are essential sources of energy in the human diet. Most of the carbohydrate in food comes from plants, which convert sunlight into carbohydrate in a process called photosynthesis. The only significant animal sources of carbohydrate in the human diet are lactose from dairy products and fructose from honey.

Monosaccharides are carbohydrates that contain only one carbohydrate molecule. There are two different types of monosaccharide, glucose and fructose, both of which are found in fruits and vegetables. When two monosaccharides combine they form disaccharides, such as lactose, sucrose (table sugar), maltose (found in malted wheat and barley) and trehalose (found in mushrooms).

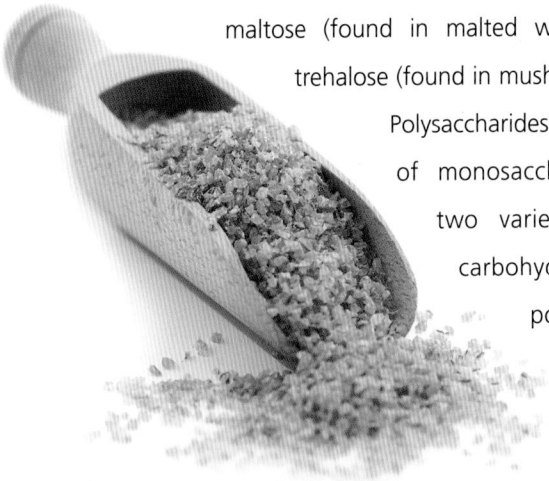

Polysaccharides are made up of chains of monosaccharides and come in two varieties: starch (complex carbohydrate) and non-starch polysaccharide (fibre). Plants store energy in the form of complex carbohydrate, which is found in large amounts in grains and roots. Fibre is found in plant cell walls where it plays a structural role.

CARBOHYDRATE DIGESTION

Glucose provides the fuel for all the body's metabolic activities. It is either absorbed directly from the digestive tract, or released from the breakdown of di- and polysaccharides into monosaccharides during digestion. Absorption is slowed by eating raw foods, starchy foods, and by the presence of protein and fats.

Carbohydrate digestion begins in the mouth where chewing breaks up the food and mixes it with a digestive enzyme called amylase. Gastric acid in the stomach breaks the food down further, but the main digestion occurs in the small intestine with the help of enzymes secreted by the pancreas.

Carbohydrate that escapes digestion in the small intestine is fermented in the large intestine, and turned into fatty acids and gas. The fatty acids are absorbed, and so is the gas to a certain extent, but if too much gas is produced it is expelled as wind. Absorbed gas is excreted through the lungs. The fermentation of small polysaccharides, such as inulin (found in dandelion root, Jerusalem artichoke, asparagus, onion and garlic) stimulates the growth of bifidobacteria, and helps to protect the natural bacterial flora of the digestive tract.

CARBOHYDRATES AND HEALTH

Simple sugars (mono- and disaccharides) are found within the cell walls of fruits and vegetables, and can also be extracted from sugar cane, sugar beet, maple, corn or honey. They are very easily absorbed into the bloodstream, and the quick energy boost they provide can seem very attractive when you are feeling low. However, an abundance of sugar in the blood is always followed by a corresponding release of insulin, which promotes the transportation of sugar into cells. This in turn causes a drop in blood-sugar levels, followed by a renewed feeling of lethargy and a craving for more sugar.

Refined sugar is a disaccharide made from sugar cane and sugar beets, leaving molasses as a by-product. It is associated with a range of health problems including tooth decay, obesity, diabetes, Crohn's disease, candida, heart disease and cancer.

The average Westerner consumes about 30 kilos (67.5 lbs) of refined sugar per year, mostly as an added ingredient in processed foods and drinks. "Raw" cane sugar is less refined and contains sucrose plus small quantities of micronutrients.

Complex carbohydrates (starch) are found in the cell walls of whole grains, vegetables and raw fruits. During digestion, cell walls are broken down to make the carbohydrate accessible for absorption. Foods rich in complex carbohydrates are good for health for four reasons: they do not expose the teeth to the effects of "free" sugars; they slow the digestive process, producing a feeling of fullness; they help to maintain stable blood-sugar levels; and their non-digestible plant cell walls (fibre) provide bulk for the faeces. Even though complex carbohydrates are made from the same building blocks as simple sugars, they release their sugar molecules at a much slower rate, producing a more measured insulin response and steadier blood-sugar and energy levels.

Fibre (non-starch polysaccharide) comes in two forms – soluble and insoluble. Soluble fibre (including pectins, gums and mucilages) is easily digested whereas insoluble fibre (including cellulose, hemicellulose and lignans) passes through the digestive tract undigested. A high intake of foods naturally rich in soluble and insoluble fibre reduces the risk of gallstones, and may also decrease the risk of coronary heart disease by lowering blood cholesterol levels. Insoluble fibre reduces the time it takes for food to pass through the gut by increasing the bulk of faeces, and helps to protect against digestive disorders and cancer. Soluble fibre protects the lining of the digestive tract and reduces the risk of blood clot formation. Foods high in fibre also tend to be rich in health-protective micronutrients, such as vitamins, antioxidants and phytochemicals, and help to improve the control of blood-sugar levels in diabetes. High-fibre diets give an average digestive "transit time" of 24 to 48 hours, compared with the average American diet, which gives an average transit time of 72 hours. A long intestinal transit time is a risk factor for diverticulitis and colon cancer.

Bran fibre (in wholemeal bread and some breakfast cereals) can, paradoxically, cause constipation because it absorbs water from the gut. If you eat a lot of bran, it is important to drink at least 1.5 litres (3 pints) of water per day to counter this effect. Eating an excess of foods with added fibre may also decrease the absorption of drugs, vitamins, minerals and other nutrients.

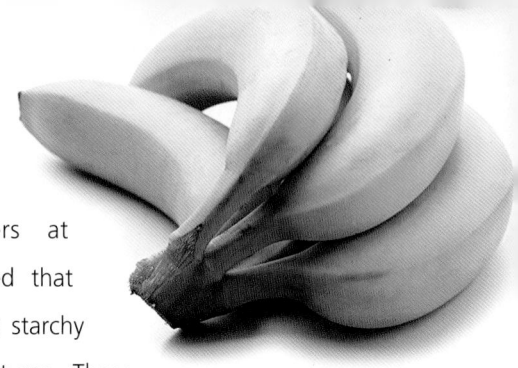

ACRYLAMIDE

In April 2002, researchers at Stockholm University reported that they had found acrylamide in starchy foods fried at high temperatures. These findings attracted worldwide attention because acrylamide is thought to be associated with cancer, neurological damage and infertility. Acrylamide is used in water purification, in the manufacture of cosmetics, plastics and other industrial products, and as an additive to commercial herbicides. It is also found in tobacco smoke. At the moment it is not understood how acrylamide is formed in foods, but it may be the result of a natural chemical reaction caused by baking or frying foods for long periods at very high temperatures. The use of grains and vegetables that have been exposed to acrylamide-containing herbicides may also be implicated.

Food safety agencies are investigating the matter further, but do not advise people to change their diet on the basis of the current evidence. Whatever risk exists can be minimized by eating plenty of fresh organic foods, and by avoiding excessive high-temperature cooking and heat-treated processed foods.

All about proteins

Between ten and fifteen per cent of the calories we consume each day come from protein. Though it can be used as an energy source, the main purpose of protein is to provide the building blocks necessary for the growth and maintenance of body structures.

Proteins are complex chemicals, which come in many shapes and sizes. They all contain amino acids linked together into chains and folded into specific shapes. Protein chains vary in length from two to thousands of amino acids. There are twenty naturally occuring amino acids, and the proteins we eat contain varying amounts of each. The body is capable of converting most amino acids from one type to another according to need, but there are eight which it cannot make. These are the essential amino acids and must be obtained from the diet.

During digestion, protein is broken down into amino acids and then absorbed in the small intestine. After absorption, amino acids are transported to the liver for processing, and then distributed in the bloodstream to become part of enzymes, body cells, hormones, hair, nails, bones, muscles and

DNA. The body is continually recombining amino acids to make new proteins, and nearly all body cells are capable of synthesizing specific proteins for their own purposes. Worn-out proteins are dismantled by the liver and excreted in the urine. The body maintains a protein reserve of between three and four hundred grams to compensate for variations in protein intake.

As mentioned earlier, the absorption of carbohydrate into the bloodstream after a meal stimulates the release of insulin from the pancreas. In addition to promoting the uptake of glucose into the body's cells, insulin encourages protein synthesis in the muscles and liver, and inhibits protein breakdown. As long as there are calories available from carbohydrate, there is no need to use body protein for energy. Unlike fat and carbohydrate, protein is used as a source of energy only under exceptional circumstances, for example, in cases of starvation, serious injury or major disease, such as cancer.

During fasting and in times of trauma or stress, another hormone called glucagon is released from the pancreas. Glucagon encourages the body to use amino acids instead of carbohydrates for fuel. The stress hormones, cortisol and adrenalin, act in a similar way, causing the protein in muscles to be broken down into free amino acids for conversion into energy. Trauma and stress can therefore cause the loss of substantial amounts of protein, especially from muscle tissue.

PROTEIN NEEDS

Nutritionists used to assume that, since protein is used to build and maintain body tissues, eating more protein must be good for us. It is now clear, however, that eating too much protein can lead to health problems, including osteoporosis and kidney disease. Human protein requirements change according to the need for growth, tissue repair, metabolism and activity, but the current consensus is that a diet containing ten per cent protein is more than adequate to maintain health. Since nearly all foods contain at least ten per cent of their calories as protein, it follows that if you satisfy your calorie needs with good quality food, you will easily meet your protein requirements. In the developed world it is rare to see anyone protein deficient.

Earlier recommendations for human protein intake differentiated between "first class" animal proteins and "second class" plant proteins, on the basis that the animal proteins had an amino acid content similar to human body proteins. It has since been established that plant-based foods, such as grains, cereals, pulses and vegetables, contain all the essential amino acids, albeit in different proportions. Far from being second class, plant proteins come packaged with other important nutrients such as fibre and phytochemicals, and are also naturally low in fat and cholesterol.

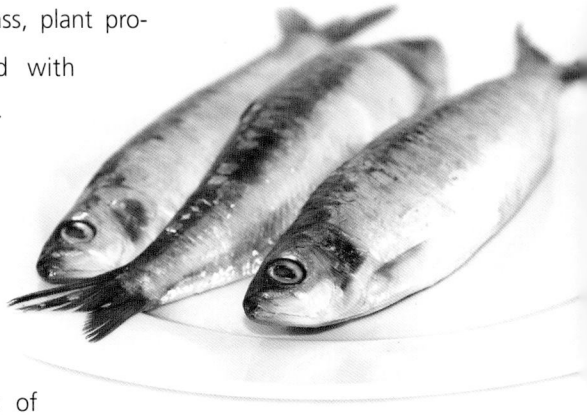

Even the concept of essential amino acids is under review, since it is now understood that some essential amino acids can be made from other precursor chemicals in the diet, and some can be synthesized in the digestive tract. Essential amino acids are also recycled from worn-out proteins before these are excreted from the body. If no protein is eaten, 90 per cent of amino acids can be recycled.

All about fats

Fats are energy-dense foods containing nine calories per gram – more than twice as much as carbohydrate or protein. They supply the body with essential fatty acids, carry fat-soluble vitamins, aid metabolism, and provide structure for cell membranes. They also make food taste good.

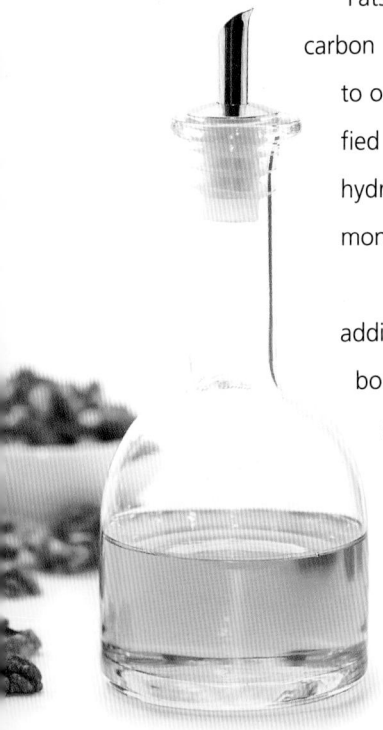

Fats contain fatty acids, which are long hydrocarbon chains with a "carboxyl group" attached to one end. There are three main types, classified according to the organization of the hydrogen atoms in their chains – saturated, monounsaturated and polyunsaturated.

Saturated fatty acids have no room for additional hydrogen atoms on their hydrocarbon chains. This makes them very stable, and solid at room temperature. They are mainly found in meat, lard, butter, cheese and milk.

Monounsaturated fatty acids have room for two extra hydrogen atoms and exist as thick oils at room temperature. Olive oil is mainly monounsaturated, and is thought to protect against heart disease by lowering blood cholesterol levels. It is the best choice for cooking because it reacts less to heat than saturated or polyunsaturated fats and oils.

Polyunsaturated fatty acids have room for more than two extra hydrogen atoms. They are sensitive to heat, light and air, and tend to go rancid unless kept in a cool, dark place. Thin vegetable oils consist mostly of polyunsaturated fat and essential fatty acids (EFAs) – so called because they cannot be made by the body and therefore must be obtained from the diet.

Essential fatty acids keep blood vessels, nerves, skin and other tissues in good condition and take part in the production of prostaglandins, which are important for normal immune function, cholesterol management and blood clotting.

The two most important EFAs are linoleic acid (an omega-6 fatty acid) and linolenic acid, which exists in two forms, gamma-linolenic acid (an omega-6 fatty acid), and alpha-linolenic acid (an omega-3 fatty acid). Omega-6 fatty acids are found in most vegetable oils and are thought to lower blood cholesterol and Low Density Lipoproteins (see opposite). Oily fish, soya beans, evening primrose oil, walnuts, flax seeds and pumpkin seeds are rich in omega-3 fatty acids, which reduce inflammation and protect the heart.

TRANS FATS

Saturated fats have a higher melting point than unsaturated fats, which makes them useful in food processing. Unsaturated fats are sometimes turned into saturated trans fats by a chemical process known as hydrogenation. Trans fats are linked to a number of health problems, including cancer, atherosclerosis and infertility. To avoid trans fats, choose products marked "no trans fats" or "unhydrogenated" whenever possible.

BODY FAT

Body fat is our energy store, which we draw on whenever our diet is lacking in calories. Excess fat and carbohydrate in the diet increases the amount of body fat, while fasting causes fat breakdown. Many drugs and toxins find their way into fatty tissues, so fasting is a powerful way to detox the body.

CHOLESTEROL AND LIPOPROTEINS

Cholesterol and steroid hormones are made from sterols. High levels of cholesterol in the blood increase the risk of cardiovascular disease. Despite its bad reputation, cholesterol is a vital component of cell membranes, and is involved in the production of bile acids and sex hormones. It is not necessary to eat cholesterol, however, because the body makes all that it needs.

Meat, eggs and dairy products tend to have a high cholesterol content. But it is not eating cholesterol per se that causes high blood cholesterol. The problem is that foods rich in cholesterol also tend to have a high saturated fat content. Excess saturated fat in the diet leads to high levels of Low Density Lipoproteins (LDLs) in the blood. Lipoproteins are fat molecules designed to transport fatty acids around the body. LDLs are the main carriers of cholesterol in the blood, and are known as "bad" lipoproteins because they are associated with high blood cholesterol levels. High Density Lipoproteins are known as "good" lipoproteins because they mop up excess cholesterol and return it to the liver for reprocessing and excretion. HDLs also remove cholesterol from clogged up arteries, helping to prevent cardiovascular disease.

FATS IN FOOD

Most foods contain at least some fat. Oily fish, vegetable oils, nuts, seeds, olives, avocados, meats, dairy products, butter and table fats are all examples of high-fat foods, but the types of fatty acids they contain vary (see lists, opposite).

Olive oil is the best known source of monounsaturated fat. Vegetable foods contain mostly polyunsaturated fat and, together with oily fish, these are the main sources of essential fatty acids in the diet.

In terms of their fat content, fish can be divided into two categories – lean and oily. Both contain monounsaturated and polyunsaturated fats. Virtually all of the fat in lean fish is found in the liver, whereas oily fish carry their fat reserves in the flesh. Oily fish and walnuts are good sources of omega-3 fatty acids.

Meat and dairy products (which contribute 23 per cent of the fat in the average Western diet) contain mostly saturated fats, and eggs contain a lot of cholesterol. However, the composition of the fat in meat and dairy products depends on the animals' diet and lifestyle. Active animals, fed on pasture and grains, have a lower saturated-fat content in their meat than those reared using intensive farming methods.

FATS IN FOODS

(Listed according to predominate fat type)

SATURATED	MONOUNSATURATED	POLYUNSATURATED
Beef	Almond oil	Brazil nuts
Burgers	Almonds	Cereals
Butter	Avocados	Corn oil
Cakes and biscuits	Fish	Evening primrose oil
Cheese	Game*	Fish
Chocolate	Hazelnuts	Grouse
Cream	Low-fat spread	Pulses
Coconut	Olive oil	Safflower oil
Eggs	Olives	Sesame oil
Hydrogenated oil	Peanuts	Sesame seeds
Ice cream		Soft vegetable margarine
Lamb		Soya beans
Lard		Soya oil
Margarine		Soya products
Milk		Sunflower oil
Palm oil		Sunflower seeds
Pork		Vegetables
Poultry		Walnut oil
Sausages		Walnuts
Suet		Wheat germ oil

*Monounsaturated fats in meat and dairy products are sometimes present in the form of trans fats which have adverse effects on health.

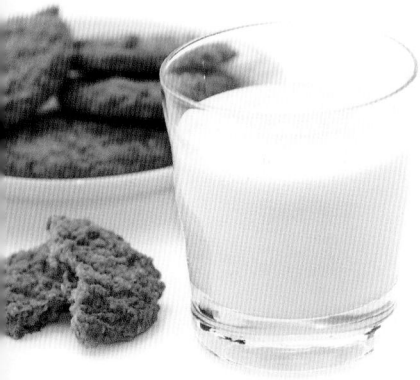

FAT GUIDELINES

- Keep your daily fat intake at or below 30 per cent of your total calorie intake.
- Keep the ratio of unsaturated to saturated fat in your diet to at least 2:1 (that is to say, eat twice as many foods containing unsaturated fats as those containing saturated fats).
- Include omega-3 fatty acids in your diet by eating walnuts, flax seeds and/or oily fish, or by taking drops of evening primrose or borage oil.
- Eat more low-fat protein foods, such as pulses, fish and poultry, and reduce the amount of red meat, offal, eggs and dairy products that you eat.
- Choose lean cuts of meat and trim off any excess fat.
- Limit the amount of fried foods you eat.
- If you eat dairy products, choose low-fat alternatives whenever possible.
- Keep foods that are rich in cholesterol (such as meat, dairy products and eggs) to a minimum in your diet.

CARBOHYDRATE, FAT AND PROTEIN TABLES

These tables provide a breakdown of the calorie, protein, carbohydrate and fat content of a wide selection of foods. The calorie content of each food is given "per average portion" to allow you to work out the calorie content of your diet without the need for using weights and measures.

The carbohydrate, protein and fat contents of each food are given as percentages of total calories. This enables you to compare the nutrient contents of foods with the Quality Calorie Targets (QCTs) for those nutrients, given at the top of the relevant columns. Total carbohydrate content is also broken down into simple sugars, complex carbohydrates and fibre, and total fat is broken down to indicate the ratio of unsaturated to saturated fat, and the amount of cholesterol and essential fatty acids ("n" is given where the figure is not known, "tr" denotes trace). In addition, a quality-calorie points score indicates which foods have the best balance of nutrients.

FRUIT

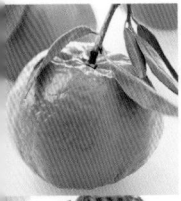

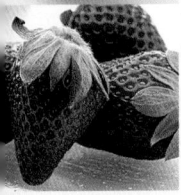

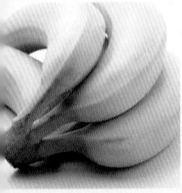

FOOD	AVERAGE PORTION SIZE	TOTAL CALORIES	PROTEIN CONTENT	
(where appropriate, numbers in brackets represent number of fruit in average portion)	grams per portion	kcals per portion	% of kcals (QCT: 10% of total kcals)	grams per portion (QCT: men 55g/day; women 45g/day)
Fresh fruit				
Apple (1)	100	**47**	3%	0.4
Apricot (2)	130	**40**	12%	1.2
Date (4)	100	**124**	5%	1.5
Fig (2)	110	**47**	12%	1.4
Grapes (bunch)	100	**60**	3%	0.4
Kiwi fruit (2)	120	**59**	9%	1.3
Melon (all types) (1 slice)	180	**43**	10%	1.1
Peach/nectarine (1)	150	**55**	13%	1.8
Pear (1)	170	**68**	3%	0.5
Plum/greengage (2)	100	**39**	7%	0.7
Rhubarb	100	**7**	51%	0.9
Sharon fruit (1)	110	**80**	4%	0.9
Tropical fruit				
Banana (1)	100	**95**	5%	1.2
Guava (1)	140	**36**	12%	1.1
Lychee (5)	75	**44**	6%	0.7
Mango (1/2)	180	**103**	5%	1.3
Papaya/paw-paw (1/4)	140	**50**	6%	0.7
Passion fruit (5)	75	**27**	29%	2.0
Pineapple (2 slices)	160	**66**	4%	0.6
Pomegranate (1)	100	**51**	10%	1.3
Citrus fruit				
Clementine/satsuma/tangerine (2)	120	**43**	10%	1.1
Grapefruit/pomelo, pink (1)	180	**54**	11%	1.4
Lemon/lime (1)	100	**12**	23%	0.8
Orange (1)	160	**59**	12%	1.8
Berries				
Blackberries (20)	100	**25**	14%	0.9
Blackcurrants	100	**28**	13%	0.9

continues

CARBOHYDRATE CONTENT				FAT CONTENT				QUALITY CALORIE POINTS
% of kcals (QCT: 60% of total kcals)	% of carbs as simple carbs	% of carbs as complex carbs	fibre in grams per portion (QCT: 16–24g/day)	% of kcals (QCT: less than 30% of total kcals)	unsat./sat. fat ratio (QCT: at least 2:1)*	cholesterol in mg per portion	EFAs in grams per portion (QCT: at least 5g/day)	max 100
95%	100%	0%	2.0	2%	n	0	n	**75**
85%	99%	1%	2.5	3%	n	0	n	**75**
94%	100%	0%	3.6	1%	n	0	n	**73**
82%	100%	0%	2.5	6%	n	0	n	**75**
96%	100%	0%	0.8	1%	n	0	n	**71**
82%	97%	3%	2.3	9%	n	0	n	**77**
86%	100%	0%	1.6	4%	n	0	n	**76**
85%	100%	0%	3.4	2%	n	0	n	**76**
95%	100%	0%	3.7	2%	n	0	n	**74**
91%	100%	0%	2.3	2%	n	0	n	**74**
43%	100%	0%	2.3	6%	n	0	n	**76**
95%	100%	0%	1.8	1%	n	0	n	**81**
92%	90%	10%	3.1	3%	n	0	n	**76**
71%	98%	2%	6.6	17%	n	0	n	**81**
92%	100%	0%	1.1	2%	n	0	n	**75**
92%	98%	2%	5.2	3%	n	0	n	**80**
91%	100%	0%	3.2	3%	n	0	n	**77**
61%	100%	0%	2.5	10%	n	0	n	**81**
92%	100%	0%	2.1	4%	n	0	n	**75**
86%	100%	0%	3.4	4%	n	0	n	**77**
87%	100%	0%	2.0	3%	n	0	n	**76**
86%	100%	0%	2.9	3%	n	0	n	**76**
58%	100%	0%	1.6	19%	n	0	n	**80**
86%	100%	0%	2.9	2%	n	0	n	**76**
79%	100%	0%	6.6	7%	n	0	n	**81**
86%	100%	0%	7.8	1%	n	0	n	**82**

**0.5 means half as much unsaturated fat as saturated fat; 2.0 means twice as much*

FRUIT

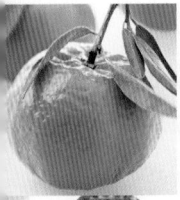

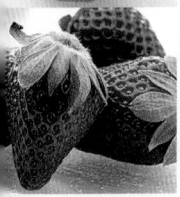

FOOD	AVERAGE PORTION SIZE	TOTAL CALORIES	PROTEIN CONTENT	
(where appropriate, numbers in brackets represent number of fruit in average portion)	grams per portion	kcals per portion	% of kcals (QCT: 10% of total kcals)	grams per portion (QCT: men 55g/day; women 45g/day)
Blueberries (bilberries)	100	**30**	8%	0.6
Cherries (10)	100	**48**	8%	0.9
Cranberries	100	**15**	11%	0.4
Elderberries	100	**35**	8%	0.7
Gooseberries	100	**40**	6%	0.7
Raspberries (25)	100	**25**	22%	1.4
Redcurrants	100	**21**	21%	1.1
Strawberries (10)	120	**32**	12%	1.0
Dried fruit				
Apricot (10)	100	**132**	10%	3.4
Date (6)	100	**203**	5%	2.5
Fig (5)	100	**227**	6%	2.2
Pear (10 slices)	100	**207**	3%	0.8
Pineapple (6 slices)	100	**276**	4%	1.3
Prune (10)	100	**160**	7%	1.4
Raisins/sultanas (3 tbs)	100	**163**	3%	1.3

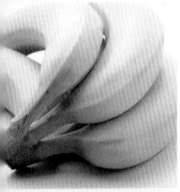

CARBOHYDRATE CONTENT				FAT CONTENT				QUALITY CALORIE POINTS
% of kcals (QCT: 60% of total kcals)	% of carbs as simple carbs	% of carbs as complex carbs	fibre in grams per portion (QCT: 16–24g/day)	% of kcals (QCT: less than 30% of total kcals)	unsat./sat. fat ratio (QCT: at least 2:1)*	cholesterol in mg per portion	EFAs in grams per portion (QCT: at least 5g/day)	max 100
86%	100%	0%	2.5	6%	n	0	n	**87**
90%	100%	0%	0.2	2%	n	0	n	**75**
83%	100%	0%	3.8	6%	n	0	n	**80**
79%	100%	0%	n	13%	n	0	n	**80**
84%	100%	0%	3.1	10%	n	0	n	**77**
67%	100%	0%	6.7	11%	n	0	n	**83**
78%	100%	0%	7.4	1%	n	0	n	**82**
85%	100%	0%	2.4	3%	n	0	n	**79**
87%	100%	0%	15.1	3%	n	0	n	**88**
94%	100%	0%	5.9	1%	n	0	n	**76**
88%	100%	0%	7.4	6%	n	0	n	**79**
95%	100%	0%	10.8	2%	n	0	n	**74**
92%	100%	0%	4.4	4%	n	0	n	**75**
90%	100%	0%	7.3	3%	n	0	n	**78**
96%	100%	0%	3.7	1%	n	0	n	**71**

**0.5 means half as much unsaturated fat as saturated fat; 2.0 means twice as much*

NUTS AND SEEDS

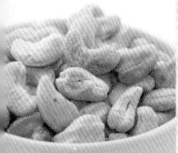

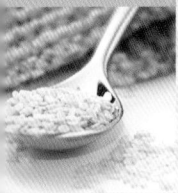

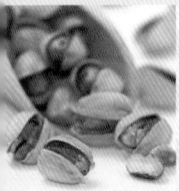

FOOD	AVERAGE PORTION SIZE	TOTAL CALORIES	PROTEIN CONTENT	
	grams per portion	kcals per portion	% of kcals (QCT: 10% of total kcals)	grams per portion (QCT: men 55g/day; women 45g/day)
Almonds	50	**306**	14%	10.6
Brazil nuts	50	**341**	8%	7.1
Cashew nuts	50	**287**	12%	8.9
Chestnuts, dried	50	**160**	5%	1.9
Coconut, fresh	100	**351**	4%	3.2
Coconut, desiccated	50	**302**	4%	2.8
Hazelnuts	50	**325**	9%	7.1
Macadamia nuts (salted)	50	**374**	4%	4.0
Melon seeds	50	**292**	20%	14.3
Peanuts	50	**282**	18%	12.8
Peanut butter	20	**125**	15%	4.5
Pecan nuts	50	**345**	5%	4.6
Pine nuts	50	**344**	8%	7.0
Pistachio nuts (salted)	50	**301**	12%	9.0
Pumpkin seeds	50	**285**	17%	12.2
Sesame seeds	50	**299**	12%	9.1
Sesame spread (tahini)	50	**304**	12%	9.3
Sunflower seeds	50	**291**	14%	9.9
Walnuts	50	**344**	9%	7.4

CARBOHYDRATE CONTENT				FAT CONTENT				QUALITY CALORIE POINTS
% of kcals (QCT: 60% of total kcals)	% of carbs as simple carbs	% of carbs as complex carbs	fibre in grams per portion (QCT: 16–24g/day)	% of kcals (QCT: less than 30% of total kcals)	unsat./sat. fat ratio (QCT: at least 2:1)*	cholesterol in mg per portion	EFAs in grams per portion (QCT: at least 5g/day)	max 100
4%	61%	39%	6.5	82%	10.3	0	7.1	**71**
2%	77%	23%	4.1	90%	3.0	0	11.5	**64**
12%	25%	75%	1.6	76%	3.9	0	4.4	**67**
81%	19%	81%	5.8	14%	4.4	0	1.1	**77**
4%	100%	0%	12.2	92%	0.1	0	0.8	**47**
4%	100%	0%	10.6	92%	0.1	0	0.8	**48**
3%	67%	33%	4.5	88%	11.9	0	3.0	**63**
3%	83%	17%	2.7	93%	5.6	0	0.8	**45**
6%	n	n	n	74%	2.9	0	13.1	**69**
8%	50%	50%	3.7	74%	4.3	0	7.2	**68**
7%	51%	49%	1.4	78%	3.4	0	3.7	**59**
3%	74%	26%	2.4	92%	10.7	0	9.4	**66**
2%	97%	3%	1.0	90%	13.3	0	20.6	**74**
5%	69%	31%	3.1	83%	6.1	0	9.0	**68**
10%	7%	93%	2.7	73%	4.2	0	9.2	**67**
1%	44%	56%	4.0	87%	5.7	0	12.8	**67**
1%	44%	56%	4.0	87%	5.7	0	12.9	**69**
12%	9%	91%	3.0	74%	9.1	0	15.5	**79**
2%	79%	21%	3.0	89%	10.7	0	23.8	**81**

**0.5 means half as much unsaturated fat as saturated fat; 2.0 means twice as much*

VEGETABLES AND PULSES

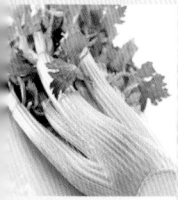

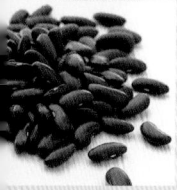

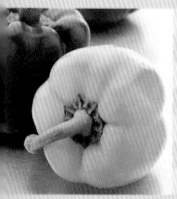

FOOD	AVERAGE PORTION SIZE	TOTAL CALORIES	PROTEIN CONTENT	
	grams per portion	kcals per portion	% of kcals (QCT: 10% of total kcals)	grams per portion (QCT: men 55g/day; women 45g/day)
Root vegetables				
Beetroot	100	**36**	19%	1.7
Carrot	100	**35**	7%	0.6
Celeriac	100	**18**	29%	1.2
Parsnip	100	**64**	11%	1.8
Potato, baked	180	**245**	11%	7.0
Potato, boiled in salted water	180	**130**	10%	3.2
Potato, mashed	180	**187**	7%	3.2
Potato, chips (all types, average)	180	**398**	6%	6.1
Swede	100	**24**	12%	0.7
Sweet potato, baked	130	**150**	6%	2.1
Beans, peas and lentils				
Aduki beans, cooked	100	**123**	30%	9.3
Baked beans, in tomato sauce	130	**105**	24%	6.2
Bean sprouts, fresh	60	**19**	37%	1.7
Black gram, blackeye, mung (av.)	100	**99**	33%	8.1
Broad beans, fresh	120	**71**	39%	6.8
Butter beans, cooked	100	**103**	28%	7.1
Chick peas, cooked	100	**121**	28%	8.4
Green beans, fresh	100	**24**	32%	1.9
Haricot beans, cooked	100	**95**	28%	6.6
Lentils, cooked (all types, average)	100	**105**	34%	8.8
Peas, fresh	100	**83**	33%	6.9
Pinto beans, cooked	100	**137**	27%	8.9
Red kidney beans, cooked	100	**103**	33%	8.4
Runner beans, fresh	100	**22**	29%	1.6
Soya beans, cooked	100	**141**	40%	14.0
Tempeh (fermented soya bean)	100	**166**	50%	20.7
Tofu (soya bean curd)	100	**73**	44%	8.1

continues

CARBOHYDRATE CONTENT				FAT CONTENT				QUALITY CALORIE POINTS
% of kcals (QCT: 60% of total kcals)	% of carbs as simple carbs	% of carbs as complex carbs	fibre in grams per portion (QCT: 16–24g/day)	% of kcals (QCT: less than 30% of total kcals)	unsat./sat. fat ratio (QCT: at least 2:1)*	cholesterol in mg per portion	EFAs in grams per portion (QCT: at least 5g/day)	max 100
78%	97%	3%	2.8	3%	n	0	n	**80**
85%	96%	4%	2.6	8%	n	0	n	**75**
50%	78%	22%	5.1	21%	n	0	n	**80**
74%	48%	52%	4.3	15%	n	0	n	**81**
88%	4%	96%	4.9	1%	6.0	0	0.1	**79**
89%	4%	96%	2.5	1%	6.0	0	0.1	**76**
56%	6%	94%	2.3	37%	n	0	n	**74**
54%	2%	98%	5.4	40%	n	0	n	**61**
77%	98%	2%	2.4	11%	6.7	0	0.2	**80**
91%	52%	48%	3.9	3%	1.0	0	0.3	**72**
69%	2%	98%	11.1	1%	n	0	n	**85**
69%	38%	62%	8.6	7%	3.8	0	0.4	**79**
48%	55%	45%	3.4	15%	n	0	n	**82**
62%	1%	99%	5.3	5%	n	0	n	**86**
46%	19%	81%	7.3	15%	n	0	n	**87**
67%	9%	91%	4.6	5%	n	0	n	**81**
56%	6%	94%	5.1	16%	n	0	n	**83**
49%	72%	28%	3.0	19%	n	0	n	**82**
67%	6%	94%	22.9	5%	n	0	n	**91**
60%	2%	98%	3.8	6%	n	0	n	**83**
51%	25%	75%	4.7	16%	1.0	0	tr	**73**
67%	n	n	n	6%	n	0	n	**85**
63%	6%	94%	9.0	4%	n	0	n	**89**
55%	88%	12%	2.6	16%	11.0	0	0.1	**84**
13%	52%	48%	6.1	47%	n	0	n	**76**
15%	16%	84%	4.1	35%	n	0	n	**78**
4%	50%	50%	0.3	52%	n	0	n	**77**

**0.5 means half as much unsaturated fat as saturated fat; 2.0 means twice as much*

VEGETABLES AND PULSES

FOOD	AVERAGE PORTION SIZE	TOTAL CALORIES	PROTEIN CONTENT	
(where appropriate, numbers in brackets represent number of vegetables in average portion)	grams per portion	kcals per portion	% of kcals (QCT: 10% of total kcals)	grams per portion (QCT: men 55g/day; women 45g/day)
Miscellaneous vegetables				
Artichoke hearts (2)	100	**18**	62%	2.8
Asparagus (5 spears)	125	**31**	46%	3.6
Aubergine (½)	130	**20**	24%	1.2
Avocado (1)	145	**276**	4%	2.8
Broccoli, green/purple	100	**34**	49%	4.2
Brussels sprouts (9)	100	**42**	33%	3.5
Cabbage (all types, average)	100	**26**	26%	1.7
Cauliflower	100	**34**	42%	3.6
Celery (3 sticks)	100	**7**	29%	0.5
Courgette	100	**18**	40%	0.9
Cucumber (5 cm chunk)	120	**12**	28%	0.4
Curly kale	100	**33**	41%	3.4
Endive	100	**13**	55%	1.8
Fennel	100	**12**	30%	0.9
Lettuce (all types, average)	80	**10**	30%	0.7
Mushrooms, common	100	**13**	55%	1.8
Mushrooms, shiitake	50	**28**	12%	0.8
Okra	100	**31**	36%	2.8
Olive (10)	30	**31**	3%	0.3
Onion/leek (all types, average)	100	**28**	19%	1.3
Pepper, green/red (½)	80	**19**	15%	0.7
Pumpkin	180	**23**	22%	1.3
Seaweed, dried (all types, average)	10	**8**	80%	1.7
Spinach	100	**25**	45%	2.8
Spring greens	100	**33**	36%	3.0
Sweetcorn	100	**93**	15%	3.4
Swiss chard	100	**19**	38%	1.8
Tomato (1)	85	**14**	16%	0.6
Watercress	80	**18**	54%	2.4

CARBOHYDRATE CONTENT				FAT CONTENT				QUALITY CALORIE POINTS
% of kcals (QCT: 60% of total kcals)	% of carbs as simple carbs	% of carbs as complex carbs	fibre in grams per portion (QCT: 16–24g/day)	% of kcals (QCT: less than 30% of total kcals)	unsat./sat. fat ratio (QCT: at least 2:1)*	cholesterol in mg per portion	EFAs in grams per portion (QCT: at least 5g/day)	max 100
28%	98%	2%	n	10%	n	0	n	**78**
30%	95%	5%	2.1	24%	n	0	n	**79**
55%	91%	9%	3.0	21%	n	0	n	**85**
4%	98%	2%	4.9	92%	7.1	0	2.8	**65**
24%	92%	8%	4.2	27%	n	0	n	**72**
37%	79%	21%	3.8	30%	n	0	n	**79**
59%	98%	2%	2.9	15%	n	0	n	**85**
33%	86%	14%	1.9	25%	n	0	n	**74**
48%	99%	1%	1.6	23%	n	0	n	**82**
37%	94%	6%	0.9	23%	1.3	0	tr	**68**
52%	93%	7%	0.8	20%	n	0	n	**78**
16%	93%	7%	3.3	43%	5.5	0	0.3	**72**
29%	99%	1%	2.0	16%	n	0	n	**73**
56%	94%	6%	2.4	14%	n	0	n	**75**
37%	99%	1%	1.0	33%	n	0	n	**74**
12%	50%	50%	2.3	33%	2.5	0	0.3	**64**
83%	n	n	n	5%	n	0	n	**80**
36%	83%	17%	4.5	28%	n	0	n	**78**
1%	tr	0%	1.2	96%	5.8	0	0.4	**53**
76%	96%	4%	2.2	5%	n	0	n	**80**
70%	98%	2%	1.5	15%	4.0	0	0.2	**82**
63%	85%	15%	0.9	15%	n	0	n	**84**
tr	-	-	5.0	20%	n	0	n	**65**
24%	94%	6%	3.9	31%	5.5	0	0.3	**75**
35%	87%	13%	6.1	28%	5.5	0	0.3	**78**
68%	12%	88%	3.3	17%	4.9	0	1.9	**83**
57%	21%	79%	n	5%	5.5	0	0.3	**85**
69%	99%	1%	1.1	15%	n	0	n	**82**
7%	98%	2%	2.4	39%	n	0	n	**65**

**0.5 means half as much unsaturated fat as saturated fat; 2.0 means twice as much*

VEGETABLE DISHES

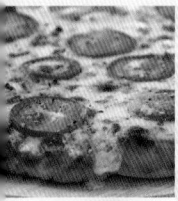

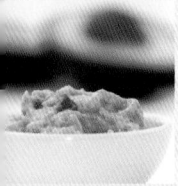

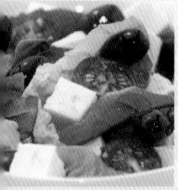

FOOD (where appropriate, numbers in brackets represent number of items in average portion)	AVERAGE PORTION SIZE grams per portion	TOTAL CALORIES kcals per portion	PROTEIN CONTENT % of kcals (QCT: 10% of total kcals)	PROTEIN CONTENT grams per portion (QCT: men 55g/day; women 45g/day)
Bakes and flans				
Cannelloni	200	**290**	12%	8.7
Casserole, bean and vegetable	250	**115**	24%	7.0
Cauliflower cheese	200	**210**	23%	12.1
Flan, vegetable	120	**253**	10%	6.4
Lasagne, vegetable	450	**527**	16%	21.6
Moussaka, vegetable	350	**480**	13%	16.1
Nut roast	150	**528**	15%	20.0
Pizza, cheese and tomato	300	**711**	15%	27.3
Shepherd's pie, vegetable	300	**339**	16%	13.8
Burgers, cutlets and pancakes				
Beanburger (no bun)	75	**152**	12%	4.7
Dosa with vegetable filling (1)	200	**307**	15%	11.6
Falafel (3)	100	**179**	14%	6.4
Nut cutlet (2)	120	**347**	7%	5.8
Onion bhaji/pakora (1)	50	**156**	6%	2.3
Pancake with vegetable filling (1)	200	**298**	11%	8.2
Quorn (myco-protein)	100	**86**	55%	11.8
Samosa, vegetable (1)	100	**217**	9%	5.1
Tempeh burger (1)	60	**116**	16%	4.6
Tofu burger (1)	60	**71**	28%	4.9
Vegeburger (1)	60	**147**	26%	9.5
Curries, stews and rice dishes				
Bhaji, cauliflower	250	**535**	7%	10.0
Bhaji, mushroom	250	**415**	4%	4.3
Bhaji, potato	250	**395**	6%	5.8
Broccoli in cheese sauce	200	**236**	22%	13.0
Bubble and squeak	200	**248**	5%	2.8
Curry, cauliflower and potato	250	**148**	23%	8.5
Curry, chick pea and spinach	250	**498**	12%	15.0

continues

CARBOHYDRATE CONTENT				FAT CONTENT				QUALITY CALORIE POINTS
% of kcals (QCT: 60% of total kcals)	% of carbs as simple carbs	% of carbs as complex carbs	fibre in grams per portion (QCT: 16–24g/day)	% of kcals (QCT: less than 30% of total kcals)	unsat./sat. fat ratio (QCT: at least 2:1)*	cholesterol in mg per portion	EFAs in grams per portion (QCT: at least 5g/day)	max 100
33%	19%	81%	2.0	55%	1.5	30	4.6	**70**
63%	49%	51%	5.5	13%	4.0	0	0.8	**86**
19%	58%	42%	2.8	58%	0.9	26	2.6	**61**
36%	13%	87%	2.0	54%	1.8	12	4.8	**75**
43%	33%	67%	7.2	41%	1.0	27	2.3	**70**
25%	29%	71%	5.6	62%	2.1	91	9.8	**77**
19%	17%	83%	8.1	66%	5.2	0	11.3	**83**
40%	9%	91%	5.7	45%	1.1	66	6.3	**75**
52%	9%	91%	7.8	32%	8.0	0	5.7	**92**
40%	20%	80%	4.6	48%	7.3	0	3.8	**75**
42%	14%	86%	6.0	43%	8.0	0	6.8	**78**
33%	17%	83%	4.4	53%	8.4	0	5.3	**68**
24%	7%	93%	3.2	69%	7.4	0	12.6	**68**
27%	15%	85%	3.5	67%	7.9	0	3.6	**67**
39%	26%	74%	2.4	50%	1.9	60	5.0	**68**
9%	55%	45%	4.8	36%	n	n	n	**78**
52%	9%	91%	n	39%	n	0	n	**76**
46%	5%	95%	1.3	38%	5.8	0	1.7	**64**
42%	21%	79%	1.3	30%	4.8	0	1.1	**62**
11%	45%	55%	2.2	63%	n	n	n	**49**
7%	80%	20%	5.5	86%	7.7	0	9.9	**76**
10%	68%	32%	5.0	86%	7.9	0	7.8	**75**
39%	9%	91%	4.0	55%	8.2	0	4.7	**85**
15%	54%	46%	3.0	63%	0.8	42	2.0	**56**
29%	14%	86%	3.8	66%	7.5	0	8.6	**70**
42%	39%	61%	4.8	35%	5.7	0	2.8	**82**
24%	7%	93%	10.8	64%	7.8	0	17.3	**91**

**0.5 means half as much unsaturated fat as saturated fat; 2.0 means twice as much*

VEGETABLE DISHES

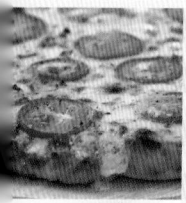

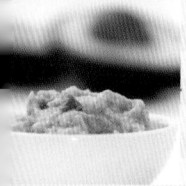

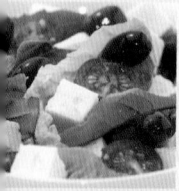

FOOD	AVERAGE PORTION SIZE	TOTAL CALORIES	PROTEIN CONTENT	
(where appropriate, numbers in brackets represent number of items in average portion)	grams per portion	kcals per portion	% of kcals (QCT: 10% of total kcals)	grams per portion (QCT: men 55g/day; women 45g/day)
Curry, red lentil and mung bean	250	**285**	17%	12.0
Curry, red lentil and tomato	250	**230**	14%	8.0
Curry, okra	250	**273**	10%	6.5
Curry, mixed vegetable	250	**123**	11%	3.5
Okra with tomato and onion	250	**450**	6%	7.3
Ratatouille	250	**205**	6%	3.3
Risotto (brown rice)	350	**501**	11%	14.4
Side dishes, dips, spreads and sauces				
Guacamole	100	**128**	4%	1.4
Houmous	60	**112**	16%	4.6
Laverbread	100	**52**	25%	3.2
Pesto sauce	25	**129**	16%	5.1
Red cabbage, stewed with apple	100	**59**	6%	0.9
Tofu spread	50	**104**	9%	2.3
Vegetable pâté	50	**87**	17%	3.8
Vegetable stir-fry	100	**64**	13%	2.0
Vine leaves, stuffed with rice (3)	100	**262**	4%	2.8
Salads				
Coleslaw, with vinaigrette	100	**87**	5%	1.1
Salad, bean, with vinaigrette	100	**147**	11%	4.2
Salad, beetroot, with vinaigrette	100	**100**	8%	2.0
Salad, carrot, nut, with vinaigrette	100	**218**	4%	2.1
Salad, Greek	100	**130**	8%	2.7
Salad, green (no dressing)	100	**12**	23%	0.7
Salad, pasta, veg., with mayonnaise	100	**127**	8%	2.6
Salad, potato, with vinaigrette	100	**157**	4%	1.5
Salad, potato, with mayonnaise	100	**239**	3%	1.6
Salad, Waldorf	100	**193**	3%	1.4
Tabouleh orientale	100	**119**	9%	2.6

CARBOHYDRATE CONTENT				FAT CONTENT				QUALITY CALORIE POINTS
% of kcals (QCT: 60% of total kcals)	% of carbs as simple carbs	% of carbs as complex carbs	fibre in grams per portion (QCT: 16–24g/day)	% of kcals (QCT: less than 30% of total kcals)	unsat./sat. fat ratio (QCT: at least 2:1)*	cholesterol in mg per portion	EFAs in grams per portion (QCT: at least 5g/day)	max 100
32%	9%	91%	5.5	51%	7.9	0	8.0	**86**
34%	29%	71%	4.8	52%	7.5	0	6.5	**88**
18%	77%	23%	9.0	72%	7.0	0	10.3	**83**
52%	52%	48%	4.0	37%	2.2	0	2.0	**79**
11%	82%	18%	11.5	83%	5.3	0	5.3	**80**
18%	84%	16%	5.0	76%	7.3	0	8.5	**81**
49%	14%	86%	12.6	40%	5.7	0	8.8	**98**
7%	59%	41%	2.6	89%	3.5	0	1.5	**56**
23%	17%	83%	1.9	61%	n	0	n	**73**
11%	tr	100%	2.8	64%	n	0	n	**74**
1%	75%	25%	n	83%	2.5	11	2.5	**51**
51%	94%	6%	2.7	43%	2.9	0	1.2	**76**
4%	67%	33%	0.3	87%	5.5	0	5.8	**64**
13%	3%	97%	n	70%	n	tr	n	**64**
38%	61%	39%	n	50%	6.0	0	2.1	**76**
34%	44%	56%	2.9	62%	5.6	0	2.2	**66**
54%	98%	2%	1.9	41%	6.4	0	2.3	**80**
33%	20%	80%	3.7	56%	7.6	0	4.2	**78**
31%	90%	10%	2.0	61%	8.1	0	3.2	**75**
23%	96%	4%	3.2	73%	8.8	0	5.8	**78**
6%	100%	tr	1.1	86%	2.6	9	1.3	**54**
57%	94%	6%	1.2	20%	10.0	0	0.1	**84**
39%	17%	83%	2.1	53%	5.4	6	4.3	**71**
33%	7%	93%	1.3	63%	7.8	0	5.1	**80**
19%	9%	91%	1.1	78%	5.6	20	12.0	**71**
14%	99%	1%	1.7	83%	6.3	13	10.7	**71**
54%	4%	96%	n	37%	8.8	0	2.0	**86**

**0.5 means half as much unsaturated fat as saturated fat; 2.0 means twice as much*

MEAT AND MEAT DISHES

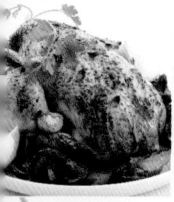

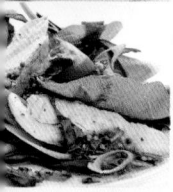

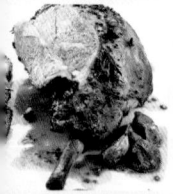

FOOD	AVERAGE PORTION SIZE	TOTAL CALORIES	PROTEIN CONTENT	
	grams per portion	kcals per portion	% of kcals (QCT: 10% of total kcals)	grams per portion (QCT: men 55g/day; women 45g/day)
Beef				
Mince	200	**458**	40%	46.2
Roast	120	**341**	33%	28.1
Steak	120	**295**	47%	17.5
Veal cutlet	150	**323**	58%	47.1
Lamb				
Chop	160	**443**	27%	29.3
Cutlet	100	**244**	25%	15.2
Roast	120	**319**	39%	31.3
Pork				
Bacon	100	**477**	20%	24.1
Chop	120	**395**	19%	19.1
Roast	120	**343**	38%	32.3
Poultry and game				
Chicken, roast	120	**259**	42%	27.1
Duck, roast	120	**407**	23%	23.5
Goose, roast	120	**383**	37%	35.2
Grouse, roast	120	**208**	72%	37.6
Hare/rabbit, roast or stewed	120	**230**	62%	35.9
Partridge, roast	120	**254**	69%	44.0
Pheasant, roast	120	**256**	61%	38.6
Pigeon, roast	120	**276**	48%	33.4
Turkey, roast	120	**205**	66%	33.6
Venison, roast or stewed	120	**238**	71%	42.0
Offal				
Heart (all types, average)	100	**208**	55%	18.0
Kidney (all types, average)	100	**160**	62%	24.9
Liver (all types, average)	100	**213**	44%	24.2
Oxtail	100	**243**	50%	30.5
Tripe	150	**150**	59%	22.2

continues

CARBOHYDRATE CONTENT				FAT CONTENT				QUALITY CALORIE POINTS
% of kcals (QCT: 60% of total kcals)	% of carbs as simple carbs	% of carbs as complex carbs	fibre in grams per portion (QCT: 16–24g/day)	% of kcals (QCT: less than 30% of total kcals)	unsat./sat. fat ratio (QCT: at least 2:1)*	cholesterol in mg per portion	EFAs in grams per portion (QCT: at least 5g/day)	max 100
0%	-	-	0	60%	1.2	164	1.2	**53**
0%	-	-	0	67%	1.2	98	1.0	**44**
0%	-	-	0	53%	1.2	98	0.7	**48**
8%	n	n	n	34%	1.2	89	0.5	**52**
0%	-	-	0	73%	0.9	176	1.7	**44**
0%	-	-	0	75%	0.9	110	1.0	**42**
0%	-	-	0	61%	0.9	132	1.0	**44**
	-	-						
0%	-	-	0	80%	1.3	80	3.1	**46**
0%	-	-	0	81%	1.3	132	2.2	**47**
0%	-	-	0	62%	1.6	132	1.8	**49**
0%	-	-	0	58%	1.8	120	2.5	**52**
0%	-	-	0	77%	2.4	192	4.2	**55**
0%	-	-	0	63%	n	n	n	**53**
0%	-	-	0	28%	3.0	n	3.7	**61**
0%	-	-	0	38%	1.3	85	3.0	**55**
0%	-	-	0	31%	2.7	n	2.0	**56**
0%	-	-	0	39%	1.8	n	1.4	**54**
0%	-	-	0	52%	n	n	n	**54**
0%	-	-	0	34%	1.7	96	2.5	**57**
0%	-	-	0	29%	n	n	n	**57**
0%	-	-	0	45%	0.9	240	0.8	**45**
0%	-	-	0	38%	0.9	670	0.7	**40**
0%	-	-	0	46%	1.3	322	1.6	**55**
0%	-	-	0	50%	1.2	110	0.5	**46**
0%	-	-	0	41%	0.7	240	0.1	**40**

**0.5 means half as much unsaturated fat as saturated fat; 2.0 means twice as much*

MEAT AND MEAT DISHES

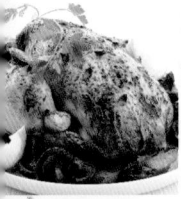

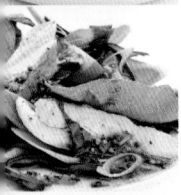

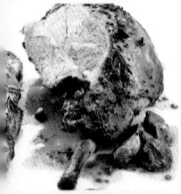

FOOD	AVERAGE PORTION SIZE	TOTAL CALORIES	PROTEIN CONTENT	
(where appropriate, numbers in brackets represent number of items in average portion)	grams per portion	kcals per portion	% of kcals (QCT: 10% of total kcals)	grams per portion (QCT: men 55g/day; women 45g/day)
Cold meats				
Corned beef	25	**54**	50%	6.7
Ham	25	**30**	62%	4.6
Luncheon meat	25	**78**	16%	3.2
Tongue	25	**53**	30%	4.0
Burgers and sausages				
Beef burger, quarterpounder	80	**211**	31%	16.3
Liver sausage (1)	50	**155**	17%	6.5
Salami (2 slices)	34	**167**	16%	6.6
Sausage (all types, average) (1)	50	**157**	13%	5.0
Turkey burger/escalope	90	**119**	90%	26.8
Meat dishes				
Black pudding	75	**229**	17%	9.7
Bolognese sauce	220	**306**	23%	17.6
Chicken chow mein	350	**515**	24%	29.8
Cornish pasty	155	**515**	10%	12.4
Haggis	100	**310**	14%	10.7
Hot pot	330	**376**	33%	30.7
Irish stew	330	**409**	17%	17.2
Lamb curry	330	**528**	23%	31.7
Lasagne	350	**669**	20%	34.3
Moussaka	330	**644**	19%	30.7
Pork pie	150	**564**	10%	14.7
Samosa (lamb)	100	**578**	5%	6.4
Sausage roll	60	**287**	6%	4.3
Shepherd's pie/cottage pie	300	**357**	26%	22.8
Shish kebab (in pitta with salad)	270	**419**	34%	36.5
Spring roll	100	**242**	11%	6.5
Steak and kidney pie	200	**646**	12%	18.6
Tandoori chicken	350	**749**	51%	95.9

CARBOHYDRATE CONTENT				FAT CONTENT				QUALITY CALORIE POINTS
% of kcals (QCT: 60% of total kcals)	% of carbs as simple carbs	% of carbs as complex carbs	fibre in grams per portion (QCT: 16–24g/day)	% of kcals (QCT: less than 30% of total kcals)	unsat./sat. fat ratio (QCT: at least 2:1)*	cholesterol in mg per portion	EFAs in grams per portion (QCT: at least 5g/day)	max 100
0%	-	-	0	50%	1.2	21	0.1	**44**
0%	-	-	0	38%	1.5	8	0.1	**47**
7%	n	n	n	77%	1.5	13	0.6	**46**
0%	-	-	0	70%	1.4	38	0.3	**44**
10%	n	n	n	59%	1.2	54	0.6	**46**
5%	n	n	n	78%	1.5	60	1.0	**47**
1%	n	n	n	83%	1.3	27	1.2	**39**
10%	n	n	n	77%	1.1	25	0.9	**45**
0%	-	-	0	10%	1.7	56	0.4	**54**
18%	n	n	n	65%	n	51	n	**56**
7%	n	n	n	70%	2.0	55	5.7	**66**
32%	4%	96%	3.9	44%	4.8	46	6.3	**78**
35%	n	n	n	55%	n	76	n	**69**
23%	n	n	n	63%	n	91	n	**62**
34%	n	n	n	33%	1.2	83	0.6	**58**
30%	n	n	n	53%	1.0	116	1.1	**57**
18%	n	n	n	59%	2.0	83	10.0	**70**
29%	19%	81%	2.8	51%	1.2	91	4.9	**70**
19%	n	n	n	62%	1.7	132	10.3	**72**
25%	n	n	n	65%	n	78	n	**61**
12%	n	n	n	83%	n	30	n	**44**
26%	n	n	n	68%	1.4	12	2.4	**44**
28%	n	n	n	46%	1.3	75	1.2	**59**
42%	11%	89%	2.7	24%	1.4	89	1.4	**65**
28%	13%	87%	1.9	61%	3.1	7	4.8	**62**
11%	n	n	n	37%	1.2	250	4.4	**64**
4%	50%	50%	tr	45%	2.1	420	7.0	**63**

**0.5 means half as much unsaturated fat as saturated fat; 2.0 means twice as much*

FISH AND FISH DISHES

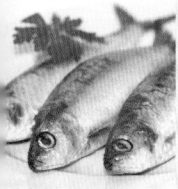

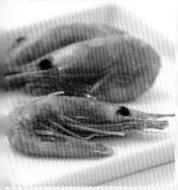

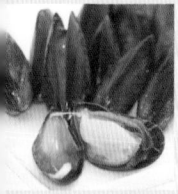

FOOD	AVERAGE PORTION SIZE	TOTAL CALORIES	PROTEIN CONTENT	
	grams per portion	kcals per portion	% of kcals (QCT: 10% of total kcals)	grams per portion (QCT: men 55g/day; women 45g/day)
White fish				
Cod, fried in batter	120	**239**	39%	23.5
Cod, grilled	120	**114**	88%	25.0
Haddock, fried	120	**209**	49%	25.7
Lemon sole, steamed	120	**109**	91%	24.7
Plaice, fried in batter	120	**308**	24%	18.3
Skate, fried in batter	120	**202**	35%	17.6
Oily fish				
Anchovies, canned	15	**29**	53%	3.8
Herring, grilled	120	**217**	44%	24.1
Kipper, grilled	120	**306**	32%	24.1
Mackerel, smoked	150	**531**	21%	28.4
Pilchards, in tomato sauce	50	**72**	46%	8.4
Salmon, canned	50	**77**	61%	11.8
Salmon, grilled	100	**215**	45%	24.2
Salmon, smoked	50	**71**	72%	12.7
Sardines, canned	100	**172**	50%	21.5
Trout, grilled	120	**162**	64%	25.8
Tuna, canned	100	**99**	95%	23.5
Seafood				
Lobster, boiled	90	**93**	86%	19.9
Mussels, boiled	40	**42**	64%	6.7
Prawns, boiled	60	**59**	91%	13.6
Shrimps, canned	50	**47**	89%	10.4
Squid, fried in batter	65	**127**	24%	7.5
Fish products and dishes				
Cod roe, fried	120	**242**	41%	25.1
Fish fingers	60	**143**	24%	8.5
Pasta with seafood	250	**275**	32%	22.3
Taramasalata	50	**252**	3%	1.6

CARBOHYDRATE CONTENT				FAT CONTENT				QUALITY CALORIE POINTS
% of kcals (QCT: 60% of total kcals)	% of carbs as simple carbs	% of carbs as complex carbs	fibre in grams per portion (QCT: 16–24g/day)	% of kcals (QCT: less than 30% of total kcals)	unsat./sat. fat ratio (QCT: at least 2:1)*	cholesterol in mg per portion	EFAs in grams per portion (QCT: at least 5g/day)	max 100
15%	n	n	tr	46%	8.1	59	9.0	**65**
0%	-	-	0	12%	1.3	49	0.4	**53**
8%	n	n	tr	43%	2.0	56	0.3	**56**
0%	-	-	0	9%	5.0	88	0.4	**59**
18%	1%	99%	0.6	58%	7.9	n	9.8	**64**
11%	1%	99%	0.2	54%	8.1	n	5.6	**61**
0%	-	-	0	47%	4.4	9	0.3	**50**
0%	-	-	0	56%	2.5	52	2.8	**58**
0%	-	-	0	68%	4.6	84	5.0	**61**
0%	-	-	0	79%	3.4	158	9.5	**61**
3%	8%	92%	tr	51%	3.3	28	1.7	**56**
0%	-	-	0	39%	3.3	14	1.0	**54**
0%	-	-	0	55%	4.0	60	4.1	**63**
0%	-	-	0	28%	3.9	18	0.7	**53**
0%	-	-	0	50%	n	60	n	**56**
0%	-	-	0	36%	3.4	84	2.0	**58**
0%	-	-	0	5%	1.5	51	0.2	**54**
tr	-	-	0	14%	4.5	99	0.5	**57**
13%	tr	tr	0	23%	2.8	23	0.4	**60**
0%	-	-	0	9%	2.0	168	0.1	**51**
tr	-	-	0	11%	3.5	65	0.2	**54**
30%	14%	86%	0.3	46%	3.3	94	2.4	**58**
6%	1%	99%	0.1	53%	6.1	378	6.8	**65**
24%	n	n	0.4	52%	2.8	19	2.8	**52**
26%	21%	79%	1	42%	0.5	103	0.8	**53**
3%	1%	99%	tr	94%	11.2	13	8.4	**64**

**0.5 means half as much unsaturated fat as saturated fat; 2.0 means twice as much*

DAIRY PRODUCTS

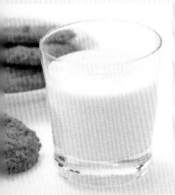

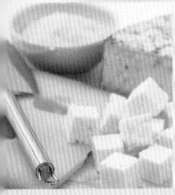

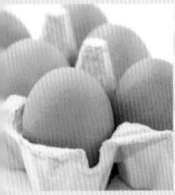

FOOD	AVERAGE PORTION SIZE	TOTAL CALORIES	PROTEIN CONTENT	
	grams/ml per portion	kcals per portion	% of kcals (QCT: 10% of total kcals)	grams per portion (QCT: men 55g/day; women 45g/day)
Milk				
Skimmed milk	200	**64**	43%	6.8
Semi-skimmed milk	200	**92**	30%	6.8
Whole milk	200	**132**	20%	6.6
Goat's milk	200	**124**	20%	6.2
Soya milk, unsweetened	200	**52**	37%	4.8
Milkshake, thick	200	**176**	17%	7.4
Cream				
Single cream	30	**58**	7%	1.0
Double cream	30	**149**	1%	0.5
Crème fraîche	30	**113**	2%	0.7
Cheeses				
Brie/camembert	40	**137**	24%	8.1
Cheddar	40	**166**	24%	10.2
Cottage cheese	40	**40**	50%	5.0
Cream cheese	40	**176**	3%	1.2
Danish blue	40	**137**	24%	8.2
Edam	40	**136**	31%	10.7
Feta	40	**100**	25%	6.2
Goat's cheese, soft	40	**128**	27%	8.4
Gouda	40	**151**	27%	10.1
Mozzarella, fresh	40	**103**	29%	7.4
Parmesan, fresh	40	**166**	35%	14.5
Stilton	40	**164**	23%	9.5
Yogurt				
Whole-milk yogurt, plain	150	**119**	29%	8.6
Greek-style yogurt, plain	150	**200**	17%	8.6
Greek-style yogurt, sheep's milk	150	**138**	21%	7.2
Soya yogurt, with fruit	150	**110**	12%	3.2
Fromage frais, plain	100	**113**	22%	6.1

continues

CARBOHYDRATE CONTENT				FAT CONTENT					QUALITY CALORIE POINTS
% of kcals (QCT: 60% of total kcals)	% of carbs as simple carbs	% of carbs as complex carbs	fibre in grams per portion (QCT: 16–24g/day)	% of kcals (QCT: less than 30% of total kcals)	unsat./sat. fat ratio (QCT: at least 2:1)*	cholesterol in mg per portion	trans fats in grams per portion (QCT: 0)	EFAs in grams per portion (QCT: at least 5g/day)	max 100
51%	100%	0%	0	6%	1.0	6	tr	tr	**70**
38%	100%	0%	0	32%	0.4	12	0.2	tr	**60**
26%	100%	0%	0	54%	0.4	28	0.2	0.2	**53**
27%	100%	0%	0	53%	0.5	22	0.2	0.4	**54**
7%	100%	0%	tr	56%	7.0	0	tr	2.2	**65**
65%	97%	3%	tr	18%	0.4	22	0.2	0.2	**57**
4%	100%	0%	0	89%	0.5	17	0.2	0.2	**40**
2%	100%	0%	0	97%	0.5	41	0.5	0.6	**32**
3%	88%	13%	0	95%	0.4	34	0.2	0.3	**35**
tr	-	-	0	76%	0.4	37	0.5	0.2	**37**
tr	-	-	0	76%	0.5	39	0.6	0.4	**37**
12%	100%	0%	0	38%	0.6	6	0.1	0.1	**47**
tr	-	-	0	97%	0.5	38	n	0.6	**34**
tr	-	-	0	76%	0.4	30	0.4	0.4	**38**
tr	-	-	0	69%	0.3	28	0.3	0.2	**35**
2%	100%	0%	0	73%	0.3	28	n	0.2	**36**
1%	100%	0%	0	72%	0.4	37	0.4	0.4	**38**
tr	-	-	0	73%	0.4	34	0.4	0.4	**37**
tr	-	-	0	71%	0.4	23	0.3	0.3	**38**
1%	100%	0%	0	64%	0.5	37	0.4	0.4	**35**
0%	-	-	0	77%	0.5	38	0.6	0.5	**35**
37%	100%	0%	n	34%	0.6	17	n	0.3	**58**
14%	94%	6%	0	69%	0.4	26	0.3	0.5	**46**
20%	100%	0%	0	59%	0.4	21	n	0.3	**49**
66%	95%	5%	0.5	22%	5.0	0	0	1.7	**80**
15%	93%	7%	0	63%	0.4	9	0.1	0.2	**48**

**0.5 means half as much unsaturated fat as saturated fat; 2.0 means twice as much*

DAIRY PRODUCTS

FOOD	AVERAGE PORTION SIZE	TOTAL CALORIES	PROTEIN CONTENT	
	grams per portion	kcals per portion	% of kcals (QCT: 10% of total kcals)	grams per portion (QCT: men 55g/day; women 45g/day)
Ice cream				
Dairy ice cream	100	**215**	7%	3.9
Non-dairy ice cream	100	**153**	8%	3.0
Eggs and egg dishes				
Egg, boiled	50	**74**	34%	6.3
Egg, fried	60	**107**	30%	8.2
Egg, scrambled	120	**308**	17%	13.1
Omelette	120	**234**	22%	13.1
Quiche	120	**378**	16%	14.9

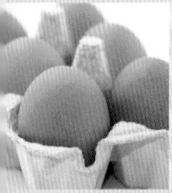

CARBOHYDRATE CONTENT				FAT CONTENT					QUALITY CALORIE POINTS
% of kcals (QCT: 60% of total kcals)	% of carbs as simple carbs	% of carbs as complex carbs	fibre in grams per portion (QCT: 16–24g/day)	% of kcals (QCT: less than 30% of total kcals)	unsat./sat. fat ratio (QCT: at least 2:1)*	cholesterol in mg per portion	trans fats in grams per portion (QCT: 0)	EFAs in grams per portion (QCT: at least 5g/day)	max 100
30%	99%	1%	tr	63%	0.5	24	0.7	0.6	**32**
46%	100%	0%	tr	46%	0.5	n	0.3	0.4	**38**
tr	-	-	0	66%	1.9	193	n	0.6	**48**
tr	-	-	0	70%	1.9	261	n	0.9	**37**
1%	100%	0%	0	82%	0.8	433	n	2.3	**48**
tr	-	-	0	78%	1.0	428	n	2.0	**36**
20%	9%	91%	0.7	64%	1.1	160	0.7	3.8	**58**

**0.5 means half as much unsaturated fat as saturated fat; 2.0 means twice as much*

FATS AND OILS

FOOD	AVERAGE PORTION SIZE	TOTAL CALORIES	PROTEIN CONTENT	
(amounts in brackets represent size of average portion)	grams/ml per portion	kcals per portion	% of kcals (QCT: 10% of total kcals)	grams per portion (QCT: men 55g/day; women 45g/day)
Cooking fats (1 tbs)				
Ghee, butter	15	**135**	tr	-
Ghee, vegetable	15	**134**	tr	-
Lard	15	**134**	tr	-
Suet, beef	15	**124**	tr	-
Suet, vegetable	15	**125**	tr	-
Table fats (on 1 slice bread)				
Butter	10	**74**	tr	-
Spread (eg. Clover)	10	**68**	tr	-
Low-fat spread (eg. Anchor)	10	**39**	7%	-
Margarine, hard (eg. Stork)	10	**72**	tr	-
- hard veg. (eg. Tomor)	10	**74**	tr	-
- polyunsat. (eg. Blue Band)	10	**75**	tr	-
Spread (70–80% fat, eg. Flora)	10	**64**	tr	-
- (60% fat, eg. Vitalite Light)	10	**55**	tr	-
- with olive oil (eg. Bertolli)	10	**57**	tr	-
- (35–40% fat, eg. Gold Sunflower)	10	**37**	5%	-
- (20–25% fat, eg. Outline)	10	**25**	10%	-
Oils (1 tbs)				
Cod liver oil	15	**135**	tr	-
Corn oil	15	**135**	tr	-
Evening primrose oil	15	**135**	tr	-
Grapeseed oil	15	**135**	tr	-
Olive oil	15	**135**	tr	-
Safflower oil	15	**135**	tr	-
Sesame oil	15	**135**	tr	-
Sunflower oil	15	**135**	tr	-
Vegetable oil, blended	15	**135**	tr	-
Walnut oil	15	**135**	tr	-
Wheat germ oil	15	**135**	tr	-

CARBOHYDRATE CONTENT			FAT CONTENT					QUALITY CALORIE POINTS
% of kcals (QCT: 60% of total kcals)	% of carbs as simple carbs	% of carbs as complex carbs	% of kcals (QCT: less than 30% of total kcals)	unsat./sat. fat ratio (QCT: at least 2:1)*	cholesterol in mg per portion	trans fats in grams per portion (QCT: 0)	EFAs in grams per portion (QCT: at least 5g/day)	max 100
tr	-	-	100%	0.4	42	n	0.5	**26**
tr	-	-	100%	1.0	0	1%	1.5	**33**
0%	-	-	100%	1.3	14	tr	1.5	**33**
5%	2%	98%	95%	0.7	12	5%	0.3	**30**
5%	0%	100%	95%	0.9	0	25%	1.9	**35**
tr	-	-	100%	0.4	23	4%	0.3	**28**
1%	100%	0%	99%	1.8	7	13%	0.9	**38**
tr	-	-	93%	1.1	5	12%	0.7	**52**
1%	100%	0%	99%	1.2	29	15%	0.5	**34**
1%	100%	0%	99%	1.2	2	18%	0.9	**35**
tr	-	-	100%	3.7	tr	8%	3.6	**58**
tr	-	-	100%	4.3	tr	4%	3.3	**50**
1%	100%	0%	99%	4.1	tr	5%	2.9	**50**
1%	100%	0%	99%	4.3	0	10%	1.3	**45**
2%	68%	32%	93%	3.1	tr	2%	1.8	**50**
4%	99%	1%	86%	2.7	1	10%	0.5	**51**
0%	-	-	100%	3.7	86	tr	4.5	**48**
0%	-	-	100%	5.6	0	tr	7.7	**54**
0%	-	-	100%	11.2	0	tr	11.5	**58**
0%	-	-	100%	7.6	0	tr	10.2	**54**
0%	-	-	100%	5.7	0	tr	1.2	**42**
0%	-	-	100%	8.9	0	tr	11.1	**57**
0%	-	-	100%	5.5	0	tr	6.5	**52**
0%	-	-	100%	7.0	0	tr	9.5	**55**
0%	-	-	100%	8.0	0	tr	7.2	**54**
0%	-	-	100%	9.5	0	tr	10.5	**56**
0%	-	-	100%	4.1	0	tr	9.1	**53**

**0.5 means half as much unsaturated fat as saturated fat; 2.0 means twice as much*

GRAINS, CEREALS, BREADS

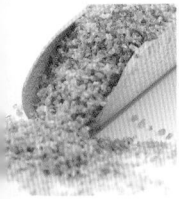

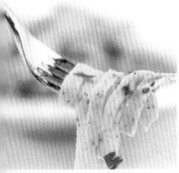

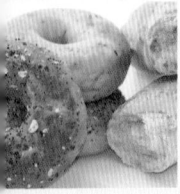

FOOD	AVERAGE PORTION SIZE	TOTAL CALORIES	PROTEIN CONTENT	
	grams per portion	kcals per portion	% of kcals (QCT: 10% of total kcals)	grams per portion (QCT: men 55g/day; women 45g/day)
Flours and grains				
Barley, pearl	100	**360**	9%	7.9
Buckwheat	100	**364**	9%	8.1
Bulgur wheat	100	**353**	11%	9.7
Cornflour	100	**354**	1%	0.6
Couscous	100	**227**	10%	5.7
Custard powder	100	**354**	1%	0.6
Millet	100	**354**	7%	5.8
Oatmeal	100	**401**	12%	12.4
Quinoa	100	**309**	18%	13.8
Rice, brown	200	**282**	7%	5.2
Rice, white	200	**276**	8%	5.2
Rice flour	100	**366**	7%	6.4
Rye flour	100	**335**	10%	8.2
Soya flour	100	**447**	33%	36.8
Wheat flour, white	100	**341**	11%	9.4
Wheat flour, wholemeal	100	**310**	16%	12.7
Wheat germ	25	**76**	35%	6.7
Wheat bran	15	**31**	27%	2.1
Noodles and pasta (cooked)				
Noodles, egg	300	**186**	14%	6.6
Noodles, plain	300	**186**	15%	7.2
Pasta, white	300	**312**	14%	10.8
Pasta, wholemeal	300	**339**	17%	14.1
Pastry				
Puff pastry	100	**373**	6%	5.7
Shortcrust pastry	100	**449**	5%	5.7
Breakfast cereals				
All-bran	50	**126**	24%	7.6
Coco pops	50	**193**	5%	2.7

continues

CARBOHYDRATE CONTENT				FAT CONTENT				QUALITY CALORIE POINTS
% of kcals (QCT: 60% of total kcals)	% of carbs as simple carbs	% of carbs as complex carbs	fibre in grams per portion (QCT: 16–24g/day)	% of kcals (QCT: less than 30% of total kcals)	unsat./sat. fat ratio (QCT: at least 2:1)*	cholesterol in mg per portion	EFAs in grams per portion (QCT: at least 5g/day)	max 100
87%	tr	100%	5.9	4%	3.1	0	0.8	**75**
87%	tr	100%	2.1	4%	n	0	n	**71**
81%	n	n	n	8%	n	0	n	**74**
97%	tr	100%	0.1	2%	4.9	0	0.3	**65**
85%	n	n	n	5%	n	0	n	**75**
97%	tr	100%	0.1	2%	n	0	n	**64**
79%	n	n	n	14%	n	0	n	**72**
68%	tr	100%	6.3	20%	4.4	0	3.5	**87**
67%	11%	89%	5.3	15%	n	0	n	**85**
86%	2%	98%	7.6	7%	n	0	n	**90**
84%	tr	100%	3.0	8%	3.2	0	0.2	**76**
82%	100%	0%	2.0	11%	n	0	n	**72**
85%	100%	0%	11.7	5%	4.3	0	1.0	**83**
20%	48%	52%	11.2	47%	2.7	0	3.3	**79**
85%	2%	98%	3.1	4%	4.1	0	0.5	**74**
78%	3%	97%	9.0	6%	3.9	0	0.9	**85**
56%	36%	64%	3.9	9%	n	0	n	**95**
49%	14%	86%	5.9	24%	3.9	0	0.4	**78**
79%	2%	98%	3.0	7%	1.2	90	1.8	**70**
79%	2%	98%	3.6	6%	n	0	n	**83**
80%	2%	98%	5.4	6%	3.8	0	0.4	**79**
77%	6%	94%	12.0	6%	n	0	n	**89**
37%	2%	98%	2.3	57%	n	57	n	**62**
39%	2%	98%	2.2	56%	1.4	11	3.5	**63**
64%	36%	64%	15.0	12%	3.9	0	1.5	**87**
92%	41%	59%	0.6	3%	n	n	n	**42**

**0.5 means half as much unsaturated fat as saturated fat; 2.0 means twice as much*

GRAINS, CEREALS, BREADS

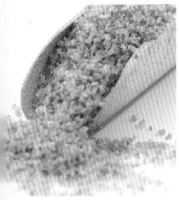

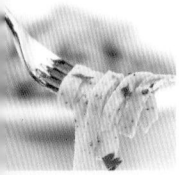

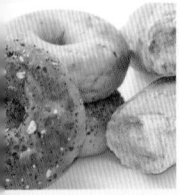

FOOD	AVERAGE PORTION SIZE	TOTAL CALORIES	PROTEIN CONTENT	
(where appropriate, numbers in brackets represent number of items in average portion)	grams per portion	kcals per portion	% of kcals (QCT: 10% of total kcals)	grams per portion (QCT: men 55g/day; women 45g/day)
Corn flakes	50	**178**	9%	4.0
Fruit 'n' Fibre	50	**176**	9%	4.1
Grapenuts	50	**173**	12%	5.3
Muesli (Swiss style)	70	**255**	12%	7.4
Porridge (made with water)	200	**98**	12%	3.0
Puffed wheat	50	**161**	18%	7.1
Rice Krispies	50	**185**	7%	3.1
Shredded wheat (2)	50	**163**	13%	5.3
Special K	50	**190**	16%	7.7
Weetabix (2)	40	**142**	12%	4.3
Breads and rolls				
Bagel (1)	90	**246**	15%	9.0
Brown bread (1 slice)	40	**87**	16%	3.4
Chapati (1)	55	**111**	14%	4.0
French baguette (5 cm slice)	40	**108**	14%	3.8
Granary bread (1 slice)	40	**94**	16%	3.7
Naan bread (1)	160	**538**	11%	14.2
Papadum (fried) (2)	26	**96**	19%	4.6
Pitta bread (1 large)	95	**252**	14%	8.7
Rye bread (1 slice)	25	**55**	15%	2.1
Wheat germ bread (1 slice)	40	**105**	14%	3.7
White bread (1 slice)	40	**94**	14%	3.4
Wholemeal bread (1 slice)	40	**86**	17%	3.7
Croissant (1)	50	**180**	9%	4.2
Hamburger bun (1)	50	**132**	14%	4.6
Morning roll (1)	50	**135**	15%	5.2
Wholemeal roll (1)	50	**121**	15%	4.5

CARBOHYDRATE CONTENT				FAT CONTENT				QUALITY CALORIE POINTS
% of kcals (QCT: 60% of total kcals)	% of carbs as simple carbs	% of carbs as complex carbs	fibre in grams per portion (QCT: 16–24g/day)	% of kcals (QCT: less than 30% of total kcals)	unsat./sat. fat ratio (QCT: at least 2:1)*	cholesterol in mg per portion	EFAs in grams per portion (QCT: at least 5g/day)	max 100
90%	8%	92%	1.7	1%	5.0	0	0.4	**69**
78%	37%	63%	5.1	13%	n	0	n	**74**
87%	15%	85%	3.1	1%	n	0	n	**73**
73%	33%	67%	5.7	15%	4.4	0	2.1	**79**
69%	tr	100%	1.6	19%	4.9	0	0.7	**73**
79%	tr	100%	4.4	4%	4.2	0	0.3	**69**
91%	12%	88%	0.6	2%	2.6	0	0.4	**69**
78%	1%	99%	5.1	8%	3.8	0	0.7	**75**
82%	22%	78%	1.4	2%	n	0	n	**72**
83%	8%	92%	3.4	5%	3.8	0	0.6	**73**
79%	11%	89%	2.2	6%	n	0	n	**71**
76%	7%	93%	2.4	8%	2.9	0	0.4	**74**
82%	4%	96%	3.5	4%	4.3	0	0.3	**75**
77%	3%	97%	2.0	9%	n	0	-	**71**
74%	5%	95%	2.6	10%	n	0	n	**75**
56%	11%	89%	3.5	33%	n	14	n	**72**
40%	0%	100%	2.4	41%	n	0	n	**53**
82%	4%	96%	3.7	4%	n	0	n	**72**
79%	4%	96%	1.5	6%	n	0	n	**73**
61%	6%	94%	2.2	25%	n	0	n	**75**
79%	5%	95%	1.5	7%	2.3	0	0.3	**70**
73%	4%	96%	3.0	10%	2.9	0	0.5	**75**
40%	3%	97%	1.3	51%	n	26	n	**61**
69%	5%	95%	2.0	17%	n	0	n	**71**
75%	4%	96%	2.1	10%	2.2	0	0.6	**71**
75%	3%	97%	4.4	10%	2.9	0	0.7	**76**

**0.5 means half as much unsaturated fat as saturated fat; 2.0 means twice as much*

BISCUITS, CAKES, PUDDINGS

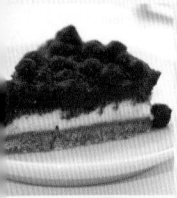

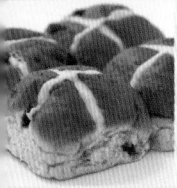

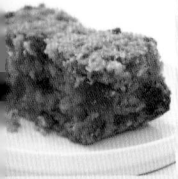

FOOD	AVERAGE PORTION SIZE	TOTAL CALORIES	PROTEIN CONTENT	
(where appropriate, numbers in brackets represent number of items in average portion)	grams per portion	kcals per portion	% of kcals (QCT: 10% of total kcals)	grams per portion (QCT: men 55g/day; women 45g/day)
Biscuits				
Chocolate biscuit (1)	25	**131**	4%	1.4
Cream cracker (1)	15	**66**	9%	1.4
Crispbread, rye (1)	10	**32**	12%	0.9
Digestive biscuit, plain (1)	15	**71**	5%	0.9
Flapjack (1)	60	**290**	4%	2.7
Wholemeal biscuit (1)	15	**54**	15%	2.0
Oatcake (1)	15	**66**	9%	1.5
Rich tea/Marie biscuit (1)	10	**46**	6%	0.7
Shortbread (1)	15	**75**	5%	0.9
Water biscuit (1)	10	**44**	10%	1.1
Wholemeal cracker (1)	15	**62**	10%	1.5
Cakes				
Chocolate cake (1 slice)	70	**319**	6%	5.2
Fruit cake (1 slice)	70	**248**	6%	3.6
Gâteau (1 slice)	70	**236**	7%	4.0
Sponge cake (1 slice)	70	**321**	6%	4.5
Swiss roll (1 slice)	35	**97**	10%	2.5
Puddings				
Cheesecake (1 slice)	110	**452**	5%	5.9
Christmas pudding	100	**291**	6%	4.6
Fruit crumble	170	**337**	4%	3.4
Custard (made with milk)	150	**176**	13%	5.6
Fruit pie	120	**223**	4%	2.4
Pancake (1)	110	**331**	8%	6.5
Rice pudding	200	**178**	15%	6.8
Trifle	170	**272**	9%	6.1
Buns and pastries				
Crumpet (1)	40	**71**	14%	2.4
Currant bun (1)	60	**178**	10%	4.6

continues

CARBOHYDRATE CONTENT				FAT CONTENT				QUALITY CALORIE POINTS
% of kcals (QCT: 60% of total kcals)	% of carbs as simple carbs	% of carbs as complex carbs	fibre in grams per portion (QCT: 16–24g/day)	% of kcals (QCT: less than 30% of total kcals)	unsat./sat. fat ratio (QCT: at least 2:1)*	cholesterol in mg per portion	EFAs in grams per portion (QCT: at least 5g/day)	max 100
49%	64%	36%	0.7	47%	0.6	n	0.3	**32**
58%	tr	100%	0.9	33%	n	n	n	**61**
82%	5%	95%	1.2	6%	4.1	0	0.1	**72**
55%	20%	80%	0.7	40%	n	3	n	**39**
47%	59%	41%	1.6	49%	n	n	n	**36**
63%	8%	92%	1.2	22%	n	0	n	**63**
54%	5%	95%	0.5	37%	3.4	0	0.8	**71**
61%	30%	70%	0.2	33%	1.0	0	0.2	**42**
48%	27%	73%	0.3	47%	0.6	11	0.2	**33**
64%	3%	97%	0.6	26%	n	0	n	**63**
65%	2%	98%	0.7	25%	n	0	n	**67**
42%	57%	43%	2.7	52%	0.5	85	0.6	**31**
61%	74%	26%	1.8	33%	1.6	37	1.2	**49**
48%	74%	26%	0.4	45%	n	116	n	**38**
42%	58%	42%	0.7	52%	1.6	90	2.7	**41**
76%	74%	26%	0.4	14%	n	66	n	**46**
23%	55%	45%	0.8	72%	0.8	120	2.3	**26**
64%	69%	31%	2.7	30%	1.0	49	0.7	**43**
64%	63%	37%	3.7	32%	1.6	n	1.9	**53**
52%	69%	31%	n	35%	0.6	24	0.2	**41**
58%	54%	46%	0.5	38%	n	4	n	**45**
43%	46%	54%	1.0	49%	1.1	80	1.6	**42**
59%	59%	41%	0.4	26%	n	30	n	**49**
52%	75%	25%	0.7	39%	1.0	85	0.7	**43**
81%	4%	96%	1.0	5%	n	0	n	**66**
67%	29%	71%	1.1	23%	n	10	n	**44**

**0.5 means half as much unsaturated fat as saturated fat; 2.0 means twice as much*

BISCUITS, CAKES, PUDDINGS

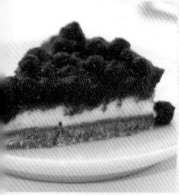

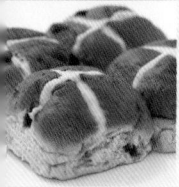

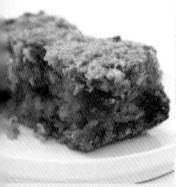

FOOD	AVERAGE PORTION SIZE	TOTAL CALORIES	PROTEIN CONTENT	
(where appropriate, numbers in brackets represent number of items in average portion)	grams per portion	kcals per portion	% of kcals (QCT: 10% of total kcals)	grams per portion (QCT: men 55g/day; women 45g/day)
Danish pastry (1)	110	**411**	6%	6.4
Doughnut (jam) (1)	75	**252**	7%	4.3
Greek pastry (Baklava) (1)	100	**322**	6%	4.7
Hot cross bun (1)	50	**155**	10%	3.7
Jam tart (1)	25	**95**	3%	0.8
Mince pie (1)	50	**212**	4%	2.2
Muffin (American)	70	**256**	7%	4.4
Muffin (English) (1)	70	**198**	14%	7.1
Scone (1)	50	**181**	8%	3.6
Teacake (1)	60	**178**	11%	4.8
Waffle (1)	65	**217**	10%	5.7

CARBOHYDRATE CONTENT				FAT CONTENT				QUALITY CALORIE POINTS
% of kcals (QCT: 60% of total kcals)	% of carbs as simple carbs	% of carbs as complex carbs	fibre in grams per portion (QCT: 16–24g/day)	% of kcals (QCT: less than 30% of total kcals)	unsat./sat. fat ratio (QCT: at least 2:1)*	cholesterol in mg per portion	EFAs in grams per portion (QCT: at least 5g/day)	max 100
52%	56%	44%	3.0	42%	n	45	n	**40**
54%	39%	61%	1.9	39%	n	11	n	**42**
46%	46%	54%	1.9	48%	n	n	n	**39**
70%	40%	60%	1.1	20%	n	13	n	**44**
62%	60%	40%	0.4	35%	1.4	2	0.5	**46**
52%	48%	52%	1.4	44%	1.5	n	1.7	**44**
54%	54%	46%	1.1	39%	0.6	48	0.6	**57**
66%	5%	95%	1.9	20%	n	21	n	**47**
56%	11%	89%	1.1	36%	1.5	3	1.1	**46**
66%	28%	72%	2.5	23%	n	11	n	**46**
45%	9%	91%	1.3	45%	n	79	n	**49**

**0.5 means half as much unsaturated fat as saturated fat; 2.0 means twice as much*

SUGAR PRODUCTS

FOOD	AVERAGE PORTION SIZE	TOTAL CALORIES	PROTEIN CONTENT	
(where appropriate, numbers in brackets represent size of average portion)	grams per portion	kcals per portion	% of kcals (QCT: 10% of total kcals)	grams per portion (QCT: men 55g/day; women 45g/day)
Sugars and syrups (1 tbs)				
Honey	20	**58**	1%	0.1
Molasses	20	**53**	0%	0
Sugar, brown	20	**72**	tr	tr
Sugar, white	20	**79**	tr	tr
Syrup, golden	20	**60**	tr	tr
Syrup, maple	20	**52**	0%	0
Treacle, black	20	**51**	2%	0.2
Preserves and spreads (1 tbs)				
Chocolate nut spread	20	**110**	5%	1.2
Fruit spread	20	**24**	3%	0.1
Jam	20	**52**	1%	0.1
Marmalade	20	**52**	tr	tr
Chocolate				
Chocolate bar (eg. Mars, Twix)	50	**221**	5%	2.7
Milk chocolate	50	**260**	6%	3.9
Plain chocolate	50	**255**	4%	2.5
Confectionery				
Boiled sweets	50	**164**	tr	tr
Cereal crunchy bar	50	**234**	9%	5.2
Fruit pastilles	50	**164**	3%	1.4
Halva (with carrot)	50	**177**	5%	2.3
Liquorice shapes	50	**139**	8%	2.8
Nougat	50	**192**	5%	2.2
Peppermints	50	**197**	1%	0.3
Turkish delight (with nuts)	50	**172**	5%	2.1

CARBOHYDRATE CONTENT				FAT CONTENT				QUALITY CALORIE POINTS
% of kcals (QCT: 60% of total kcals)	% of carbs as simple carbs	% of carbs as complex carbs	fibre in grams per portion (QCT: 16–24g/day)	% of kcals (QCT: less than 30% of total kcals)	unsat./sat. fat ratio (QCT: at least 2:1)*	cholesterol in mg per portion	EFAs in grams per portion (QCT: at least 5g/day)	max 100
98%	100%	0%	0	1%	-	0	0	**31**
97%	100%	0%	tr	3%	-	0	tr	**30**
100%	100%	0%	0	0%	-	0	0	**29**
100%	100%	0%	0	0%	-	0	0	**28**
99%	100%	0%	0	1%	-	0	0	**29**
96%	100%	0%	tr	4%	-	0	tr	**31**
98%	100%	0%	0	0%	-	0	0	**32**
41%	99%	1%	0.2	54%	2.1	tr	0.9	**39**
97%	98%	2%	n	0%	-	0	0	**36**
99%	100%	0%	0.2	0%	-	0	0	**33**
100%	100%	0%	0.1	0%	-	0	0	**33**
56%	99%	1%	n	39%	0.8	13	0.4	**37**
41%	99%	1%	0.4	53%	0.6	12	0.6	**30**
47%	98%	2%	1.3	49%	0.6	0	0.5	**33**
100%	100%	0%	0	0%	-	0	0	**29**
48%	53%	47%	n	43%	3.7	tr	2.7	**53**
97%	96%	4%	n	0%	-	0	0	**31**
47%	99%	1%	1.5	48%	0.6	25	0.7	**37**
88%	69%	31%	n	4%	n	0	n	**37**
75%	99%	1%	n	20%	6.3	0	1.4	**42**
98%	100%	0%	0	1%	n	0	n	**30**
88%	100%	0%	0.2	7%	7.0	0	0.4	**47**

**0.5 means half as much unsaturated fat as saturated fat; 2.0 means twice as much*

SOUPS AND SAUCES

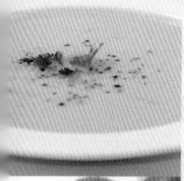

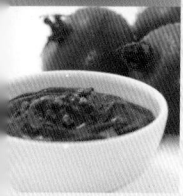

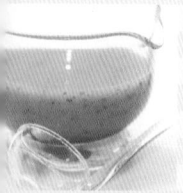

FOOD	AVERAGE PORTION SIZE	TOTAL CALORIES	PROTEIN CONTENT	
	grams/ml per portion	kcals per portion	% of kcals (QCT: 10% of total kcals)	grams per portion (QCT: men 55g/day; women 45g/day)
Soups				
Bouillabaisse	250	**338**	31%	26.0
Carrot and orange soup	250	**50**	8%	1.0
Chicken soup	250	**145**	12%	4.3
French onion soup	250	**100**	2%	0.5
Gazpacho	250	**113**	7%	2.0
Leek and potato soup	250	**130**	12%	3.8
Lentil soup	250	**293**	19%	14.0
Minestrone soup	250	**158**	11%	4.5
Mushroom soup	250	**115**	10%	2.8
Oxtail soup	250	**110**	22%	6.0
Tomato soup	250	**130**	6%	2.0
Vegetable soup	250	**130**	7%	2.3
Sauces				
Black bean sauce	30	**28**	31%	2.1
Brown sauce (spicy)	30	**36**	4%	0.4
Curry sauce	115	**90**	8%	1.7
Dressing, French	30	**139**	tr	tr
Dressing, Thousand Island	30	**97**	1%	0.3
Dressing, yogurt-based	30	**88**	3%	0.7
Gravy (instant)	70	**24**	4%	0.2
Hollandaise sauce	70	**495**	3%	3.4
Mayonnaise	30	**207**	1%	0.3
Mint sauce	10	**10**	6%	0.2
Raita	50	**29**	30%	2.2
Salad cream	30	**104**	2%	0.5
Soy sauce	10	**4**	28%	0.3
Sweet and sour sauce	150	**66**	4%	0.6
Tomato ketchup	30	**35**	6%	0.5

CARBOHYDRATE CONTENT				FAT CONTENT				QUALITY CALORIE POINTS
% of kcals (QCT: 60% of total kcals)	% of carbs as simple carbs	% of carbs as complex carbs	fibre in grams per portion (QCT: 16–24g/day)	% of kcals (QCT: less than 30% of total kcals)	unsat./sat. fat ratio (QCT: at least 2:1)*	cholesterol in mg per portion	EFAs in grams per portion (QCT: at least 5g/day)	max 100
4%	94%	6%	1.0	65%	5.6	80	2.3	**55**
69%	95%	5%	2.8	23%	2.0	0	0.3	**75**
29%	24%	76%	tr	59%	5.0	243	2.5	**62**
53%	100%	0%	3.3	45%	8.5	0	2.5	**80**
22%	96%	4%	n	71%	5.6	0	0.8	**66**
44%	24%	76%	4.5	44%	3.0	0	0.5	**75**
45%	14%	86%	6.3	36%	9.2	0	2.5	**82**
46%	18%	82%	1.5	43%	0.8	5	0.3	**61**
31%	21%	79%	0.3	59%	5.0	0	2.3	**68**
43%	18%	82%	0.3	35%	1.3	18	0.5	**62**
43%	44%	56%	1.8	51%	4.8	0	2.0	**71**
23%	56%	44%	2.8	70%	5.8	0	2.0	**66**
49%	91%	9%	0.6	20%	n	0	n	**49**
87%	87%	13%	0.2	9%	n	0	n	**42**
34%	52%	48%	n	58%	n	0	n	**34**
4%	100%	0%	0	96%	n	0	n	**36**
15%	86%	14%	0.1	84%	n	9	n	**24**
9%	75%	25%	n	88%	n	n	n	**46**
33%	3%	97%	tr	63%	n	n	n	**34**
tr	-	-	tr	97%	0.5	340	2.2	**29**
1%	76%	24%	0	98%	5.4	39	2.2	**25**
80%	100%	0%	n	14%	n	0	tr	**45**
37%	99%	1%	0.1	33%	0.6	4	0.1	**46**
18%	99%	1%	n	80%	6.6	13	5.8	**44**
71%	89%	11%	0	1%	0	0	0	**36**
90%	69%	31%	n	6%	n	0	0	**42**
93%	96%	4%	0.3	1%	n	0	tr	**42**

**0.5 means half as much unsaturated fat as saturated fat; 2.0 means twice as much*

PICKLES AND SAVOURIES

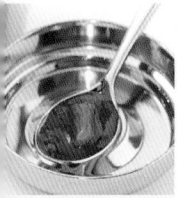

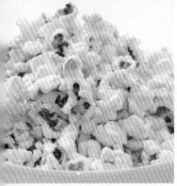

FOOD	AVERAGE PORTION SIZE	TOTAL CALORIES	PROTEIN CONTENT	
(where appropriate, numbers in brackets represent number of items in average portion)	grams per portion	kcals per portion	% of kcals (QCT: 10% of total kcals)	grams per portion (QCT: men 55g/day; women 45g/day)
Pickles and chutneys				
Lime pickle	40	**71**	4%	0.8
Piccalilli	40	**34**	5%	0.4
Relish (corn/cucumber/onion)	40	**48**	3%	0.4
Sweet mango chutney	40	**76**	2%	0.3
Tomato chutney	40	**51**	4%	0.5
Tomatoes, sun-dried	50	**248**	3%	1.7
Savoury snacks				
Bombay mix	30	**164**	15%	6.0
Breadsticks (3)	20	**78**	11%	2.2
Popcorn, plain	50	**297**	4%	3.1
Pork scratchings	25	**152**	32%	12.0
Potato crisps	40	**212**	4%	2.3
Potato crisps, low-fat	40	**183**	6%	2.6
Pretzels	50	**191**	10%	4.6
Tortilla chips	50	**230**	7%	3.8
Twiglets	50	**192**	12%	5.7

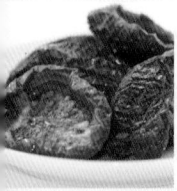

CARBOHYDRATE CONTENT				FAT CONTENT				QUALITY CALORIE POINTS
% of kcals (QCT: 60% of total kcals)	% of carbs as simple carbs	% of carbs as complex carbs	fibre in grams per portion (QCT: 16–24g/day)	% of kcals (QCT: less than 30% of total kcals)	unsat./sat. fat ratio (QCT: at least 2:1)*	cholesterol in mg per portion	EFAs in grams per portion (QCT: at least 5g/day)	max 100
18%	n	n	2.2	78%	n	0	n	**34**
78%	84%	16%	0.8	17%	4.0	0	0.1	**50**
92%	88%	12%	0.5	5%	n	0	0.1	**43**
96%	94%	6%	n	2%	n	0	tr	**44**
91%	91%	9%	0.5	5%	n	0	tr	**50**
4%	54%	46%	n	93%	6.3	0	13.6	**63**
23%	n	n	n	63%	n	0	n	**55**
70%	7%	93%	0.6	19%	0.4	0	0.2	**50**
31%	2%	98%	n	65%	8.0	0	9.9	**52**
tr	-	-	0.1	68%	n	n	n	**34**
38%	1%	99%	4.3	58%	1.0	0	2.0	**36**
52%	2%	98%	5.5	42%	1.2	0	1.0	**44**
78%	n	n	n	12%	3.3	0	0.6	**46**
49%	2%	98%	3.0	44%	4.3	0	3.4	**54**
61%	2%	98%	5.2	27%	1.3	0	0.9	**47**

**0.5 means half as much unsaturated fat as saturated fat; 2.0 means twice as much*

DRINKS

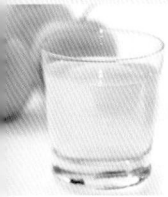

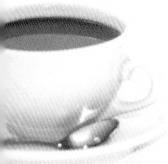

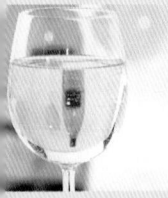

FOOD	AVERAGE PORTION SIZE	TOTAL CALORIES	ALCOHOL CONTENT	PROTEIN CONTENT	
(where appropriate, numbers in brackets represent size of average portion)	ml per portion	kcals per portion	% of kcals	% of kcals (QCT: 10% of total kcals)	grams per portion (QCT: men 55g/day; women 45g/day)
Fruit juices (unsweetened)					
Apple juice	200	**76**	0%	1%	0.2
Cranberry juice	200	**122**	0%	0%	tr
Grape juice	200	**92**	0%	3%	0.6
Grapefruit juice	200	**66**	0%	5%	0.8
Lemon juice	20	**1**	0%	17%	0.1
Lime juice	20	**2**	0%	18%	0.1
Mango juice (canned)	200	**78**	0%	1%	0.2
Orange juice	200	**66**	0%	7%	1.2
Passion fruit juice	200	**94**	0%	7%	1.6
Pineapple juice	200	**82**	0%	3%	0.6
Pomegranate juice	200	**88**	0%	2%	0.4
Prune juice	200	**114**	0%	4%	1.0
Hot drinks					
Coffee, black	190	**4**	0%	40%	0.4
Coffee, with milk	190	**13**	0%	29%	1.0
Coffee, Irish	190	**160**	43%	2%	0.8
Drinking chocolate (for 1 mug)	18	**66**	0%	6%	1.0
Horlicks (for 1 mug)	24	**95**	0%	14%	3.3
Ovaltine (for 1 mug)	24	**91**	0%	10%	2.4
Tea, black	190	**tr**	0%	tr	tr
Tea, with milk	190	**15**	0%	20%	0.8
Tea, green	190	**tr**	0%	tr	tr
Tea, herbal	190	**2**	0%	0%	0
Soft drinks (carbonated)					
Cola	330	**129**	0%	tr	n
Fruit juice drink (eg. Tango)	330	**129**	0%	tr	n
Ginger ale	250	**38**	0%	0%	0
Lemonade	200	**44**	0%	tr	tr

continues

CARBOHYDRATE CONTENT				FAT CONTENT				QUALITY CALORIE POINTS
% of kcals (QCT: 60% of total kcals)	% of carbs as simple carbs	% of carbs as complex carbs	fibre in grams per portion (QCT: 16–24g/day)	% of kcals (QCT: less than 30% of total kcals)	unsat./sat. fat ratio (QCT: at least 2:1)*	cholesterol in mg per portion	EFAs in grams per portion (QCT: at least 5g/day)	max 100
98%	100%	0%	tr	1%	n	0	n	**69**
100%	n	n	n	0%	n	0	0	**75**
95%	100%	0%	0	2%	n	0	n	**69**
94%	100%	0%	tr	1%	n	0	n	**71**
83%	100%	0%	tr	tr	n	0	n	**74**
76%	100%	0%	tr	6%	n	0	n	**75**
94%	98%	2%	tr	5%	n	0	n	**72**
92%	100%	0%	0.2	1%	n	0	n	**73**
85%	100%	0%	tr	8%	n	0	n	**76**
96%	100%	0%	tr	1%	n	0	n	**70**
97%	100%	0%	tr	1%	n	0	n	**70**
94%	100%	0%	tr	2%	n	0	n	**70**
56%	100%	0%	0	4%	n	0	tr	**59**
26%	100%	0%	0	45%	0.3	4	tr	**51**
14%	100%	0%	0	41%	0.5	40	0.4	**32**
79%	95%	5%	0	15%	n	n	n	**41**
69%	68%	32%	0	17%	n	n	n	**43**
81%	90%	10%	0	9%	n	n	n	**48**
tr	-	-	0	tr	n	0	n	**57**
23%	100%	0%	0	57%	n	4	tr	**50**
tr	-	-	0	tr	n	0	0	**69**
75%	n	n	0	25%	n	0	tr	**70**
99%	100%	0%	0	tr	n	0	0	**45**
99%	100%	0%	0	tr	n	tr	0	**46**
99%	100%	0%	0	0%	0	0	0	**45**
100%	100%	0%	0	0%	0	0	0	**45**

**0.5 means half as much unsaturated fat as saturated fat; 2.0 means twice as much*

DRINKS

FOOD	AVERAGE PORTION SIZE	TOTAL CALORIES	ALCOHOL CONTENT	PROTEIN CONTENT	
	ml per portion	kcals per portion	% of kcals	% of kcals (QCT: 10% of total kcals)	grams per portion (QCT: men 55g/day; women 45g/day)
Lucozade	200	**120**	0%	tr	tr
Tonic water	250	**83**	0%	0%	0
Soft drinks (uncarbonated)					
Barley water (diluted)	200	**28**	0%	3%	0.2
Ribena (diluted)	200	**60**	0%	tr	tr
Fruit juice drink (diluted)	200	**74**	0%	1%	0.2
Rosehip syrup (diluted)	200	**92**	0%	0%	0
Alcoholic drinks					
Beer, bitter	300	**177**	68%	4%	0.9
Beer, lager	300	**384**	96%	4%	0.9
Beer, shandy	300	**48**	30%	tr	tr
Beer, stout	300	**156**	77%	5%	1.2
Cider	300	**108**	73%	tr	tr
Champagne	125	**95**	91%	2%	0.4
Red wine	125	**85**	98%	1%	0.1
White wine	125	**83**	96%	1%	0.1
Port	50	**79**	71%	0%	0.1
Sherry	50	**58**	94%	1%	0.1
Vermouth/martini	50	**55**	90%	tr	tr
Cream liqueurs (eg. Baileys)	25	**81**	29%	tr	tr
Liqueurs, high-strength (eg. pernod)	25	**79**	71%	tr	tr
Liqueurs, med.-strength (eg. campari)	25	**66**	53%	tr	tr
Spirits (eg. brandy/gin/whisky)	25	**56**	100%	tr	tr

CARBOHYDRATE CONTENT				FAT CONTENT				QUALITY CALORIE POINTS
% of kcals (QCT: 60% of total kcals)	% of carbs as simple carbs	% of carbs as complex carbs	fibre in grams per portion (QCT: 16–24g/day)	% of kcals (QCT: less than 30% of total kcals)	unsat./sat. fat ratio (QCT: at least 2:1)*	cholesterol in mg per portion	EFAs in grams per portion (QCT: at least 5g/day)	max 100
100%	99%	1%	0	0%	0	0	0	**47**
100%	100%	0%	0	0%	0	0	0	**47**
97%	100%	0%	tr	tr	0	0	0	**47**
100%	100%	0%	0	0%	0	0	0	**47**
99%	100%	0%	tr	0%	0	0	0	**46**
100%	100%	0%	0	0%	0	0	0	**47**
27%	100%	0%	tr	1%	tr	tr	0	**32**
tr	-	-	tr	tr	tr	tr	0	**21**
70%	100%	0%	tr	0%	0	0	0	**37**
18%	100%	0%	tr	tr	tr	0	tr	**31**
27%	100%	0%	0	0%	0	0	0	**33**
7%	100%	0%	0	0%	0	0	0	**29**
1%	100%	0%	0	0%	0	0	0	**27**
3%	100%	0%	0	0%	0	0	0	**28**
29%	100%	0%	0	0%	0	0	0	**32**
5%	100%	0%	0	0%	0	0	0	**28**
10%	100%	0%	0	0%	0	0	0	**28**
26%	100%	0%	0	45%	n	n	n	**19**
29%	100%	0%	0	0%	0	0	0	**30**
47%	100%	0%	0	0%	0	0	0	**34**
tr	-	-	0	0%	0	0	0	**25**

**0.5 means half as much unsaturated fat as saturated fat; 2.0 means twice as much*

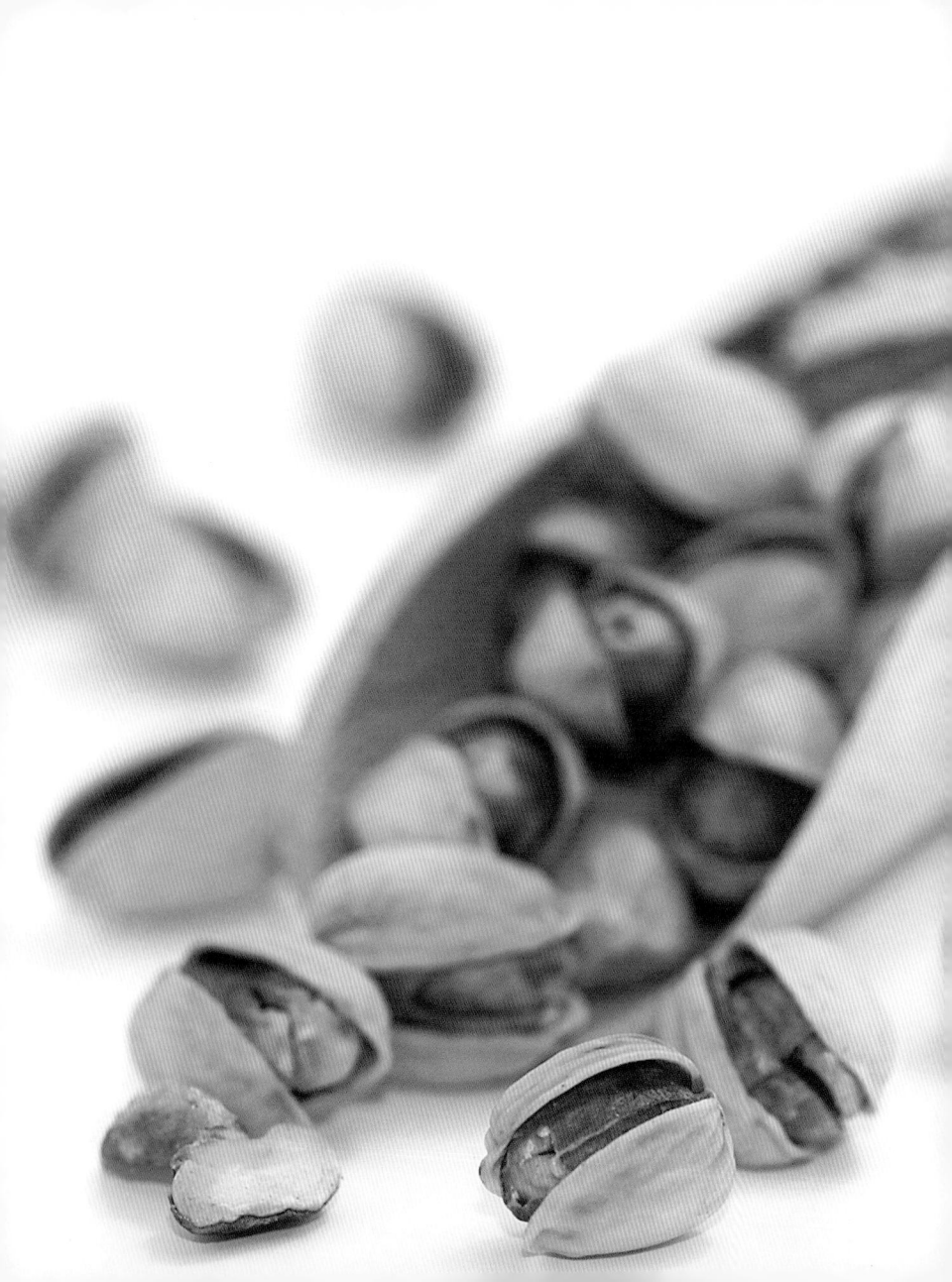

Part 3
VITAMINS, MINERALS & TRACE ELEMENTS

In this section we explore the main vitamins, minerals and trace elements that are essential to health. We look at the foods in which they can be found, how they are used within the body, the causes and symptoms of deficiency, and the effects of excessive intakes. For each nutrient there is also a box that specifies the recommended daily intake and lists the top ten foods containing that nutrient. This is followed by nutritional tables, which detail the amounts of vitamins, minerals and trace elements present in a range of foods. Using this information you can create a healthy diet that is high in essential nutrients.

All about vitamins

Fat-soluble vitamins

VITAMIN A

Vitamin A is a family of chemicals that includes retinol (derived from animal sources), and about 50 different carotenoids (derived from plant foods). The most common carotenoid is beta-carotene, which is found in abundance in carrots, green leaves and peppers. Other important carotenoids include alpha-carotene, gamma-carotene and beta-cryptoxanthin.

About one sixth of the carotenoids we eat are converted into retinol in the body and stored in the liver, fat tissues, lungs, testicles, bone marrow, eyes and kidneys. Vitamin A is important for good vision, skin, reproduction, pregnancy, growth and immunity, and also protects against bacterial, parasitic and viral infections. In addition, carotenoids are powerful antioxidants that help us resist cancer and heart disease.

The average adult needs about 500 micrograms of retinol or 3300 micrograms of beta-carotene per day. Vitamin A is found in many different foods and deficiency is rare in affluent societies, but during illness, and in cases of fat malabsorption,

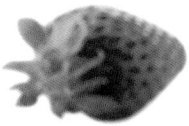

extra vitamin A (carotenoids in particular) is needed in the diet.

In poorer countries, vitamin A deficiency is a major health problem with more than 200 million children affected worldwide due to poverty, disease and severe shortages of fresh food. Vitamin A deficiency causes decreased immunity and, in severe cases, eye disease and blindness.

Taking supplements has been shown to be ineffective in the treatment of vitamin A deficiency because of problems with absorption from the digestive tract. Carotenoids in foods are well-absorbed, however. Consuming a lot of carotenoid-rich food may tint the skin yellow, but does not cause toxicity. By contrast, too much retinol can cause bone and liver damage and, in pregnancy, may harm the developing baby. Signs of retinol toxicity include headache, blurred vision, vomiting and vertigo.

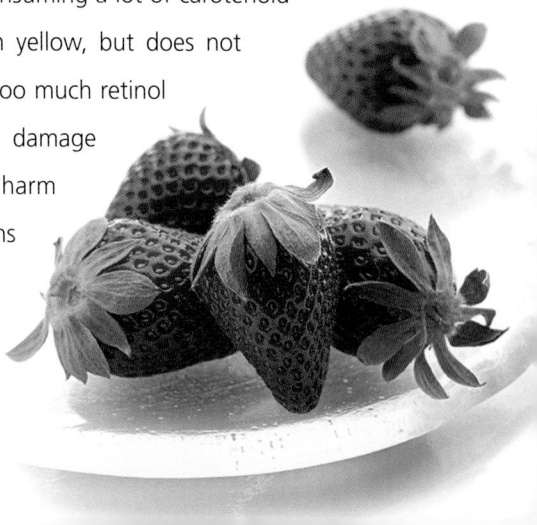

Vitamin A TOP 10 (micrograms per 100 grams of food)

BETA-CAROTENE

World Health Organisation recommended intake = 3300 µg/day

Toxicity level = none

1.	paprika	36250	6.	red pepper	3780
2.	carrots	12472	7.	spinach	3535
3.	sweet potato	8910	8.	curly kale	3145
4.	spring greens	8295	9.	watercress	2520
5.	parsley	4040	10.	canteloupe melon	1765

RETINOL

World Health Organisation recommended intake = 550 µg/day

Toxicity level = >9000 µg/day

1.	cod liver oil	18000	6.	margarine (on average)	665
2.	liver	17300	7.	crème fraîche	388
3.	liver pâté	7300	8.	cheese (on average)	300
4.	butter	958	9.	eggs	190
5.	double cream	779	10.	greek-style yogurt	115

VITAMIN D

At the beginning of the 20th century, a bone disease called rickets was rife among poor children in northern industrialized countries. It was cured – and prevented – with cod liver oil, and research revealed that this effect could be reproduced by two chemicals, cholecalciferol (Vitamin D3, found in animal tissues) and ergocalciferol (Vitamin D2, produced from plant sterols).

Many foods are now fortified with vitamin D, but sunlight is our most important source because it triggers vitamin D production in the skin. Just one hour a day of sunlight on a small patch of skin is enough, and during the summer the body produces and stores plenty to last the winter.

Vitamin D enhances calcium absorption and influences its uptake and release from bones. Deficiency causes stunted growth, bone pain and deformity, dental and nerve problems, muscle weakness, anaemia and a predisposition to respiratory infections. Too much dietary vitamin D causes abnormally high levels of calcium in the blood, leading to serious health problems, such as kidney damage. Symptoms of toxicity include loss of appetite, nausea, diarrhoea, muscle weakness and joint pain.

As most of us get sufficient vitamin D from the action of sunlight on our skin, a dietary intake is only vital for pregnant women, nursing mothers and those who are rarely exposed to sunlight, such as the housebound, the elderly, women following strict religious dress codes, submariners and astronauts.

Vitamin D TOP 10 (micrograms per 100 grams of food)

CHOLECALCIFEROL

World Health Organisation recommended intakes = 0 μg/day (if adequate exposure to sunlight), 2.5 μg/day (if no sun exposure)

Toxicity level = >50 μg/day

1.	cod liver oil	210.0	6.	kipper, mackerel	8.0
2.	herring	19.0	7.	salmon	7.1
3.	cod roe	17.0	8.	sardines, tuna	4.1
4.	trout	9.6	9.	eggs	1.8
5.	butter, lard, margarine	8.2	10.	corned beef, liver pâté	1.3

VITAMIN E

Vitamin E (also known as tocopherol) is a major antioxidant, which stabilizes cell membranes and protects them against damage from free radicals and environmental toxins. It also inhibits the production of the inflammatory prostaglandins that cause many of the symptoms of autoimmune diseases such as rheumatoid arthritis. It plays a role in the synthesis of DNA, and is thought to protect against heart disease and cancer.

Vitamin E is found in a wide variety of foods so deficiency is uncommon. However, since vitamin E has important effects on immune function, there is a distinction between the amount needed to avoid dietary deficiency and the amount needed to help prevent disease. Higher intakes (50 mg per day) can decrease the risk of immune-related conditions, and help prevent or delay the development of Parkinson's disease and other degenerative neurological disorders such as multiple sclerosis. Vitamin E is also thought to reduce the risk of cataracts, arthritis and chronic fatigue syndrome.

Vitamin E deficiency leads to cell membrane damage, which in turn causes muscle, nerve and liver dysfunction. As tobacco smoke contains large amounts of free radicals,

Vitamin E TOP 10 (milligrams per 100 grams of food)

TOCOPHEROL

World Health Organisation recommended intake = >4 mg/day

Toxicity level = >3200 mg/day

1.	wheat germ oil	136.7	6.	almonds, hazelnuts	24.5
2.	sunflower oil	49.2	7.	sundried tomatoes	24.0
3.	safflower oil	40.7	8.	wheat germ	22.0
4.	sunflower seeds	37.8	9.	cod liver oil	20.0
5.	polyunsaturated margarine	32.6	10.	corn oil	17.2

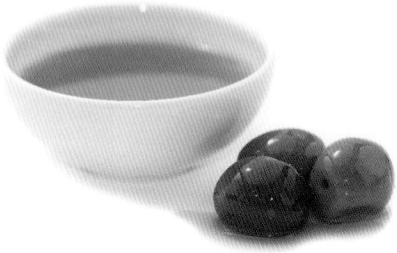

smokers should ensure their diet contains plenty of vitamin E, as should the elderly in whom increased susceptibility to illness may be related to deficiency.

When obtained from food, vitamin E has no toxic effects. However, taking high-dose vitamin E supplements may cause breast soreness, muscle weakness, psychological and gastro-intestinal disturbance and thyroid dysfunction.

VITAMIN K

There are two types of Vitamin K: phylloquinone (K1) is produced by plants involved in photosynthesis (those with green leaves); and menaquinone (K2) is produced by bacteria involved in fermentation (in foods such as cheese and tempeh). Intestinal bacteria also produce vitamin K, especially if we eat a high-fibre diet. Vitamin K is stored in the liver, and recycled many times before being broken down and excreted.

Vitamin K plays a vital role in normal blood clotting and bone health. It may help prevent osteoporosis and protect soft tissues from abnormal calcification. Deficiency is rare, but digestive diseases, such as coeliac disease, pancreatitis, cystic fibrosis and chronic liver disease, may cause deficiency since vitamin K depends on normal fat digestion for its own absorption. Symptoms of deficiency include easy bruising and bleeding, and bone fractures are also common in osteoporosis.

Haemorrhagic disease of the newborn (HDN) affects a small number of babies and was shown in the 1940s to be caused by vitamin K deficiency. Newborns used to be given protective vitamin K injections, but nowadays vitamin K is given to the mother before the birth, and to the baby by mouth once it is born. Natural vitamin K is non-toxic, even in large amounts.

Vitamin K TOP 10 (micrograms per 100 grams of food)

World Health Organisation recommended intake = 1 μg/kg/day
Toxicity level = none

1.	curly kale	623	6.	broccoli	185
2.	parsley	548	7.	brussels sprouts	153
3.	spinach	394	8.	lettuce	129
4.	watercress	315	9.	olive oil	57
5.	cabbage	242	10.	asparagus	52

Water-soluble vitamins

VITAMIN C

In the 18th century, scurvy was much feared by seafarers. The first signs were bleeding gums, leg pains, slow healing wounds and general weakness, followed by haemorrhages under the skin, swellings, ulcers and death. In 1772 James Lind (a Scottish physician) found that including citrus fruit in seamen's diets could cure scurvy in a week. Subsequent research showed that ascorbic acid, now known as vitamin C, was the key.

Vitamin C is an important antioxidant and plays a vital role in wound healing and iron absorption. It stimulates immune system cells to fight infections and helps lower blood cholesterol. It also reduces the toxic effects of radiation, and protects against serious diseases such as cancer and heart disease.

Unlike most animals, humans are unable to synthesize vitamin C, so we have to include it in our diet. Current recommended daily amounts are based on the amount necessary to protect against scurvy and promote wound healing, but many people could benefit from eating more. Animals that synthesize their own have much higher body levels of vitamin C than most humans, so it has been suggested that our vitamin C intake should be increased to produce similar levels. Cancer and rheumatoid arthritis sufferers have decreased amounts of vitamin C in their blood, as do smokers.

Today, scurvy appears only in cases of famine, severe malnutrition, malabsorption and chronic alcoholism. However, people who take more than one gram of vitamin C supplements per day can develop signs of scurvy if they suddenly reduce their intake – even though their diet provides the recommended daily amount. Very high intakes of vitamin C can cause diarrhoea and increase the risk of kidney stones.

Vitamin C TOP 10 (milligrams per 100 grams of food)

World Health Organisation recommended intake = 30 mg/day
Toxicity level = >3 g/day

1.	guava	230	6.	brussels sprouts	115
2.	blackcurrants	200	7.	curly kale	110
3.	parsley	190	8.	broccoli	87
4.	spring greens	180	9.	watercress	62
5.	green, red and chilli peppers	120	10.	papaya	60

VITAMIN B1 (THIAMIN)

Towards the end of the 19th century, an epidemic of beri-beri spread though Japan, China and South-East Asia, causing serious problems for the colonial powers with their insatiable need for cheap labour. Mortality rates exceeded 50 per cent and, although it was noticed that the disease could be cured by supplementing the staple diet of rice with fish, vegetables, meat and grains, poverty ensured that the epidemic continued. The cause of beri-beri only emerged when an "anti-beri-beri factor" (thiamin) was discovered in rice polishings – the parts of the rice grain removed during dehulling to produce polished white rice.

Vitamin B1 TOP 10 (milligrams per 100 grams of food)

THIAMIN
World Health Organisation recommended intake = 0.8 mg/day
Toxicity level = >3 g/day

1.	yeast extract	4.10	6.	pork	0.98
2.	wheat germ	2.01	7.	sesame seeds	0.94
3.	sunflower seeds	1.60	8.	oatmeal, wheat bran	0.90
4.	breakfast cereals (on average)	1.20	9.	peas	0.74
5.	peanuts	1.14	10.	brown rice	0.59

The introduction of steam-powered mills and the production of polished rice on an industrial scale had robbed the rice grain of its nutrients, and the labourers who produced it of their health.

We need vitamin B1 (thiamin) to make use of the energy contained in carbohydrates, fats and alcohol, so our daily requirement is closely linked to the amount of these foods in our diet. Foods containing carbohydrate and fat usually come ready-packed with thiamin, and a diet consisting of natural, unprocessed foods normally provides all that we need. In cereals and seeds, thiamin is found in the outer grain layers and is therefore often lost during milling and refining. To remedy this loss, many processed foods are fortified with vitamin B1.

Nowadays, vitamin B1 deficiency is associated with alcoholism, malnutrition and chronic disease. In alcoholism, symptoms of B1 deficiency include confusion and loss of memory and balance. When deficiency becomes severe, beri-beri develops, causing muscle weakness, nerve problems and eventually heart failure. Very high doses of thiamin (>3 g per day), and more moderate doses (>50 mg per day) taken over long periods, can cause toxicity symptoms, such as headaches, irritability, itching, eczema, fast pulse, sleepnessness and weakness.

VITAMIN B2 (RIBOFLAVIN)

Vitamin B2 is used in the body to release energy from proteins, fats and carbohydrates, and is found in small amounts in most foods. It is not well stored by the body, so the amount we need each day is related to how much food we eat and how many calories we spend. However much riboflavin we consume, the body only uses as much as it needs, excreting the rest in the urine. High doses of riboflavin supplements turn the urine bright yellow, but there are currently no other known side effects.

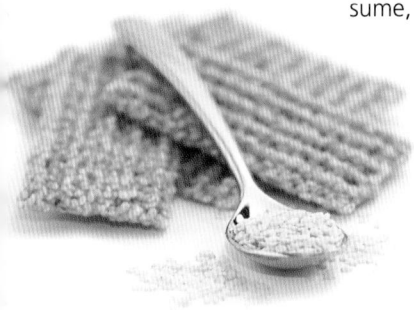

Vitamin B2 deficiency is uncommon, but those suffering from thyroid problems, diabetes, anorexia nervosa, severe malnutrition and malabsorption syndromes may become deficient. Alcohol and some drugs (including chlorpromazine and barbiturates) can also reduce vitamin B2 levels in the body. The symptoms of deficiency include cracks at the corners of the mouth, a sore tongue and a rash around the nose. Riboflavin deficiency in infancy and childhood (ariboflavinosis) leads to retarded growth.

VITAMIN B3 (NIACIN)

Vitamin B3 is actually two different chemicals, nicotinic acid and nicotinamide. They form part of a system of co-enzymes responsible for the release of energy from food. Consequently, our daily requirement for niacin depends on the amount of food we eat and how much energy we use.

Niacin is found in most foods, and the essential amino acid tryptophan (present in many protein-rich foods) can also be converted into niacin in the body. This means that as long as we eat enough protein, we naturally meet our niacin requirements.

Vitamin B2 TOP 10 (milligrams per 100 grams of food)

RIBOFLAVIN

World Health Organisation recommended intake = 1 mg/day

Toxicity level = none known

1.	yeast extract	11.90	6.	wheat germ	0.72
2.	liver, heart, kidney (on average)	2.50	7.	venison, duck, goose	0.60
3.	breakfast cereals (on average)	1.20	8.	tempeh	0.48
4.	crab	0.86	9.	eggs, cheese (on average)	0.45
5.	almonds	0.75	10.	oyster mushrooms	0.40

Vitamin B3 TOP 10 (milligrams per 100 grams of food)

NIACIN

World Health Organisation recommended intake = 14 mg/day

Toxicity level = >3 g/day

1.	yeast extract	71.0	6.	breakfast cereals (on average)	15.0
2.	wheat bran	32.6	7.	game	12.0
3.	liver	19.4	8.	sesame seeds	10.4
4.	peanuts	19.3	9.	wheat germ	9.8
5.	paprika	18.4	10.	tempeh	4.7

Apart from helping to maintain energy levels, vitamin B3 is also involved in keeping skin and mucous membranes in good condition. Deficiency is rare, and is usually only seen in cases of severe malnourishment or in those subsisting on foods low in niacin and tryptophan, such as maize or millet. It also affects alcoholics and cancer sufferers, and can be caused by a genetic defect. Symptoms of niacin deficiency (also known as pellagra) include a red skin rash, sore tongue, constipation or diarrhoea, weakness, insomnia, dementia and mental disturbance.

While pellagra responds rapidly to treatment with niacin, there is no evidence that increased intake of the vitamin is of any benefit to people without the disease. High doses can cause low blood pressure, flushing and excess stomach acid. Very high doses may also cause liver damage.

VITAMIN B5 (PANTOTHENATE)

Pantothenic means "that which is everywhere", and pantothenate, or pantothenic acid, is indeed present in almost all living tissues. It is found in most natural foods, and is produced by bacteria in the intestine. This vitamin enables the body to utilize the energy contained in fats, carbohydrates, protein and alcohol. It aids antibody production, protects against allergy

Vitamin B5 TOP 10 (milligrams per 100 grams of food)

PANTOTHENATE

World Health Organisation recommended intake = 5 mg/day

Toxicity level = none

1.	broad beans	3.8	6.	wheat bran, wheat germ	2.2
2.	offal	3.8	7.	sesame seeds	2.1
3.	breakfast cereals (on average)	3.8	8.	mushrooms	2.0
4.	peanuts	2.7	9.	eggs	1.8
5.	cod roe	2.6	10.	trout	1.6

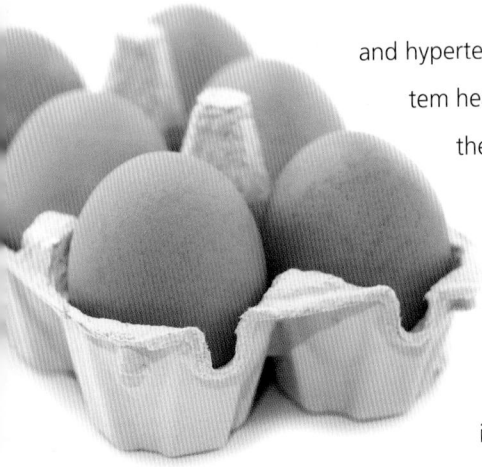

and hypertension, and maintains nervous system health. Vitamin B5 is also involved in the conversion of cholesterol into steroid hormones and in the detoxification of drugs. It is closely associated with the adrenal glands and with our ability to respond to stress, so it is also called "the stress vitamin".

Interestingly, research has shown that the ageing process may be linked to the stress response, and that older people have lower blood levels of pantothenate than younger people.

Vitamin B5 deficiency is unlikely in people who eat a diet consisting mainly of fresh foods, but in affluent societies (where many people exist on refined, canned or frozen foods, white bread and ready-made processed meals) sub-clinical pantothenate deficiency is becoming more common. Symptoms include weakness, insomnia, cramps and an increased tendency to allergy. Severe deficiency is very rare and causes pins and needles, a sensation of burning in the feet, low blood pressure and inability of the adrenal glands to respond to stress.

VITAMIN B6 (PYRIDOXINE)

Vitamin B6 was first discovered in 1934. The more protein we eat, the more vitamin B6 we need because it is involved in protein metabolism and is necessary for the conversion of tryptophan into niacin. Vitamin B6 also facilitates haemoglobin production and protects against high blood pressure and allergy. It supports the nervous and immune systems, and is used to treat nausea in early pregnancy and during radiotherapy treatment.

Vitamin B6 deficiency is uncommon, but the likelihood increases with age. It is associated with alcoholism, chronic liver and kidney disease, intestinal malabsorption disorders and

Vitamin B6 TOP 10 (milligrams per 100 grams of food)

PYRIDOXINE

World Health Organisation recommended intake = 1.3 mg/day

Toxicity level = individual tolerance varies (doses as low as 50 mg taken over long periods of time can cause neurological problems)

1.	wheat germ	3.30	6.	sesame seeds	0.76
2.	tempeh	1.86	7.	salmon	0.75
3.	muesli	1.60	8.	walnuts	0.67
4.	yeast extract	1.60	9.	venison	0.65
5.	wheat bran	1.38	10.	turkey	0.61

certain genetic disorders. It may also be linked to epilepsy, anaemia and carpal tunnel syndrome, and can be caused by the drugs used in the treatment of tuberculosis, rheumatoid arthritis and Parkinson's disease. Mild deficiency in otherwise healthy people may diminish the immune response and increase the risk of atherosclerosis and hormone-dependent cancers.

Vitamin B6 is closely involved in hormone metabolism and the menstrual cycle. Sub-clinical deficiency is relatively common in women during childbearing years, especially those who have

Vitamin B12 TOP 10 (micrograms per 100 grams of food)

COBALAMIN

World Health Organisation recommended intake = 1 μg/day

Toxicity level = none

1.	liver, kidney	58.0	6.	prawns	8.0
2.	cockles, mussels	35.0	7.	salmon, trout, mackerel	5.0
3.	nori seaweed (dried)	27.5	8.	duck, rabbit, beef, lamb, turkey, goose	2.5
4.	yeast extract, vegetable stock	13.3	9.	eggs	2.5
5.	kippers, sardines, anchovies, cod roe	11.0	10.	cheese	2.0

Breakfast cereals and vegetable margarines are often fortified with B12.

had several pregnancies or who use oral contraceptives or HRT. Pre-menstrual mood swings, acne and morning sickness – even pre-eclampsia and post-natal depression – may be related to vitamin B6 deficiency. Other symptoms include a skin rash around the eyes, nose and mouth, cracks in the corners of the mouth and the lips, a sore tongue, migraine, depression, irritability, tiredness and disturbed sensation in hands and feet.

Taking regular high doses of vitamin B6 over a long period can cause toxicity accompanied by loss of sensation in the hands and feet (which returns once intake is reduced).

VITAMIN B12 (COBALAMIN)

Vitamin B12 is produced entirely by micro-organisms living in the soil and in the intestines. It is used in DNA synthesis and is essential for all body cells, particularly blood and nerve cells. Rapidly dividing cells in the bone marrow need vitamin B12 and folic acid to produce red and white blood cells.

Vitamin B12 deficiency is rare because only tiny amounts are needed, and liver stores normally last four years. Malabsorption syndromes, intestinal parasites, alcoholism and cancer are the most likely causes of deficiency. Smoking and

Folate TOP 10 (micrograms per 100 grams of food)

World Health Organisation recommended intake = 150 μg/day
Toxicity level = none (see opposite)

1.	yeast extract	2620		broccoli	195
2.	chicken liver	1350	8.	chick peas, mung and red kidney beans	180
3.	black-eye beans	630	9.	asparagus, parsley, swiss chard, savoy cabbage	170
4.	soya flour, soya beans	345	10.	beetroot	150
5.	wheat bran	260			
6.	ox and lamb liver	250			
7.	purple-sprouting				

taking antibiotics also increase need, and strict vegetarians should include non-animal sources of B12 in their diet. Symptoms of deficiency include a sore tongue, diarrhoea and general weakness, progressing to numbness and tingling in fingers and toes, loss of balance, nerve pains and weakness in arms and legs caused by damage to the spinal cord and brain. Pernicious anaemia is a rare form of vitamin B12 deficiency caused by a lack of "intrinsic factor" – a secretion in the stomach. Without intrinsic factor, B12 cannot be absorbed.

Vitamin B12 is non-toxic, even in large doses. People suffering from malabsorption syndromes (including pernicious anaemia) usually need vitamin B12 injections.

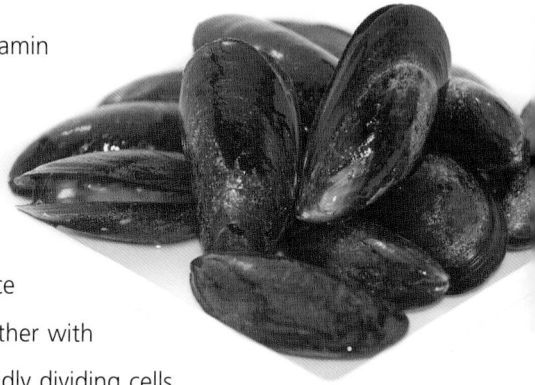

FOLATE

Folate, or folic acid, is used by the body to produce amino acids and DNA. Together with vitamin B12, it supports rapidly dividing cells and is vitally important during pregnancy for the development of the baby's nervous system. Low folate in the diet has also been linked to heart disease.

Folate deficiency has three main causes: malnourishment, particularly among the elderly, the poor and alcoholics, but also increasingly in people whose diet consists mainly of fast foods; malabsorption, caused by gastro-intestinal disease and some drugs (particularly anti-epileptic medication); and increased need (owing to pregnancy, blood disorders, cancer, AIDS and serious infection). The symptoms of deficiency include anaemia, weakness and depression. High folate intakes (usually from supplements) are not toxic, but can lead to reduced zinc absorption.

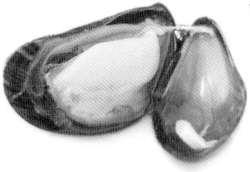

BIOTIN

Biotin is important for healthy skin, hair, sweat glands, nerves and bone marrow. It also encourages the appetite and aids fat metabolism. It is found in most foods and is manufactured by gut bacteria. Like the other B-group vitamins, it plays a role in the conversion of calories into energy.

Biotin deficiency is rare, but can be caused by poor nutrition. Symptoms include dry skin, hair loss, fatigue, nausea and lack of appetite. Severe deficiency causes muscle pains, pins and needles, anaemia and raised blood cholesterol. Biotin can be used to treat scalp conditions (such as hair loss and dandruff), skin problems (such as dry skin) and brittle nails.

Biotin TOP 10 (micrograms per 100 grams of food)

World Health Organisation recommended intake = 30 μg/day
Toxicity level = none

1.	chicken liver	216	6.	wheat bran	45
2.	peanuts	110	7.	wheat germ	25
3.	hazelnuts, almonds, soya beans	65	8.	eggs	20
4.	tempeh	53	9.	oatmeal, oatcakes	17
5.	plaice	47	10.	mushrooms	15

VITAMIN TABLES

These tables give the calorie and vitamin contents of a wide selection of foods. The vitamins are divided into fat-soluble (vitamins A, D and E) and water-soluble (vitamin C and the B-group – thiamin, riboflavin, niacin, pantothenate, pyridoxine, cobalamin, folate and biotin). The calorie and vitamin contents of each food are given "per average portion" rather than "per 100 grams". This allows you to work out the calorie and vitamin content of your diet without using weights or measures.

To find out how rich a food is in a particular vitamin, compare the amount contained in a single portion ("n" is given where the figure for a particular food is not known; "tr" denotes trace) with the Quality Calorie Target (QCT) for that nutrient, given at the top of the relevant column. This will enable you to assess your daily intake of vitamins, and help you to choose particular foods to boost your intake of certain vitamins. The figures in bold denote the foods with the highest scores for each nutrient in each food category.

FRUIT

FOOD	AVERAGE PORTION SIZE	TOTAL CALORIES	FAT-SOLUBLE VITAMINS			
			A		D	
(where appropriate, numbers in brackets represent number of fruit in average portion)	grams per portion	kcals per portion	either Retinol (µg/portion) (QCT: 550µg/day)	or Carotene (µg/portion) (QCT: 3,300µg/day)	Cholecalciferol (µg/portion) (QCT: 0µg/day*)	*(* see pages 98–9)*
Fresh fruit						
Apple (1)	100	**47**	0	18	0	
Apricot (2)	130	**40**	0	2,061	0	
Date (4)	100	**124**	0	18	0	
Fig (2)	110	**47**	0	165	0	
Grapes (bunch)	100	**60**	**41**	17	0	
Kiwi fruit (2)	120	**59**	0	44	0	
Melon (all types) (1 slice)	180	**43**	0	1,800	0	
Peach/nectarine (1)	150	**55**	0	87	0	
Pear (1)	170	**68**	0	31	0	
Plum/greengage (2)	100	**39**	0	195	0	
Rhubarb	100	**7**	0	60	0	
Sharon fruit (1)	110	**80**	0	1,045	0	
Tropical fruit						
Banana (1)	100	**95**	0	21	0	
Guava (1)	140	**36**	0	609	0	
Lychee (5)	75	**44**	0	0	0	
Mango (½)	180	**103**	0	**3,240**	0	
Papaya/paw-paw (¼)	140	**50**	0	1,134	0	
Passion fruit (5)	75	**27**	0	563	0	
Pineapple (2 slices)	160	**66**	0	29	0	
Pomegranate (1)	100	**51**	0	33	0	
Citrus fruit						
Clementine/satsuma/tangerine (2)	120	**43**	0	108	0	
Grapefruit/pomelo, pink (1)	180	**54**	0	594	0	
Lemon/lime (1)	100	**12**	0	tr	0	
Orange (1)	160	**59**	0	45	0	
Berries						
Blackberries (20)	100	**25**	0	80	0	
Blackcurrants	100	**28**	0	100	0	

continues

	WATER-SOLUBLE VITAMINS								
E	THE B-GROUP								C
Tocopherol (mg/portion) (QCT: 4mg/day)	Thiamin B1 (mg/portion) (QCT: 0.8mg/day)	Riboflavin B2 (mg/portion) (QCT: 1mg/day)	Niacin B3 (mg/portion) (QCT: 14mg/day)	Pantothenate B5 (mg/portion) (QCT: 5mg/day)	Pyridoxine B6 (mg/portion) (QCT: 1.3mg/day)	Cobalamin B12 (µg/portion) (QCT: 1µg/day)	Folate (µg/portion) (QCT: 150µg/day)	Biotin (µg/portion) (QCT: 30µg/day)	Ascorbic acid (mg/portion) (QCT: 30mg/day)
0.6	tr	tr	0.2	tr	0.1	0	1	1	12
n	0.1	0.1	0.8	0.3	0.1	0	7	n	8
n	0.1	0.1	1.4	0.2	0.1	0	25	n	14
n	tr	tr	0.7	0.2	0.1	0	n	n	2
tr	0.1	tr	0.2	0.1	0.1	0	2	0	3
n	tr	tr	0.7	0.2	0.2	0	n	n	71
0.2	0.1	tr	0.7	0.3	0.2	0	5	n	31
tr	0.1	0.1	1.4	0.2	**0.5**	0	5	0	53
0.9	tr	0.1	0.3	0.1	tr	0	3	0	10
0.7	0.1	tr	1.0	0.2	0.1	0	3	tr	5
0.2	tr	tr	0.4	0.1	n	0	7	n	6
n	tr	0.1	0.3	n	n	0	8	n	21
0.3	tr	0.1	0.9	0.4	0.3	0	14	**3**	11
0.4	0.1	0.1	1.5	0.2	0.2	0	n	n	**322**
n	tr	0.1	0.5	n	n	0	n	n	34
1.9	0.1	0.1	3.2	0.3	0.2	0	n	n	67
n	tr	0.1	0.6	0.3	tr	0	1	n	84
n	tr	0.1	1.4	n	n	0	n	n	17
0.2	0.1	0.1	0.6	0.3	0.1	0	8	0	19
n	0.1	tr	0.5	0.6	tr	0	n	n	13
n	0.1	0.1	0.5	0.2	0.1	0	40	n	44
0.3	0.1	0.1	0.7	0.5	0.1	0	47	2	73
n	tr	tr	0.3	0.2	0.1	0	10	n	50
0.4	**0.2**	0.1	0.8	0.6	0.2	0	**50**	2	86
2.4	tr	0.1	0.6	0.3	0.1	0	34	0	15
1.0	tr	0.1	0.4	0.4	0.1	0	n	2	200

FRUIT

FOOD	AVERAGE PORTION SIZE	TOTAL CALORIES	FAT-SOLUBLE VITAMINS			
			A		D	
(where appropriate, numbers in brackets represent number of fruit in average portion)	grams per portion	kcals per portion	either Retinol (µg/portion) (QCT: 550µg/day)	or Carotene (µg/portion) (QCT: 3,300µg/day)	Cholecalciferol (µg/portion) (QCT: 0µg/day*)	*(*see pages 98–9)*
Blueberries (bilberries)	100	**30**	0	30	0	
Cherries (10)	100	**48**	0	25	0	
Cranberries	100	**15**	0	22	0	
Elderberries	100	**35**	0	360	0	
Gooseberries	100	**40**	0	110	0	
Raspberries (25)	100	**25**	0	tr	0	
Redcurrants	100	**21**	0	25	0	
Strawberries (10)	120	**32**	0	tr	0	
Dried fruit						
Apricot (10)	100	**132**	0	645	0	
Date (6)	100	**203**	0	40	0	
Fig (5)	100	**227**	0	64	0	
Pear (10 slices)	100	**207**	0	91	0	
Pineapple (6 slices)	100	**276**	0	120	0	
Prune (10)	100	**160**	0	155	0	
Raisins and sultanas (3 tbs)	100	**163**	0	tr	0	

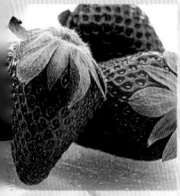

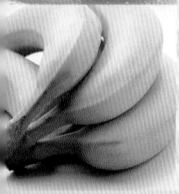

E	WATER-SOLUBLE VITAMINS								C
	THE B-GROUP								
Tocopherol (mg/portion) (QCT: 4mg/day)	Thiamin B1 (mg/portion) (QCT: 0.8mg/day)	Riboflavin B2 (mg/portion) (QCT: 1mg/day)	Niacin B3 (mg/portion) (QCT: 14mg/day)	Pantothenate B5 (mg/portion) (QCT: 5mg/day)	Pyridoxine B6 (mg/portion) (QCT: 1.3mg/day)	Cobalamin B12 (µg/portion) (QCT: 1µg/day)	Folate (µg/portion) (QCT: 150µg/day)	Biotin (µg/portion) (QCT: 30µg/day)	Ascorbic acid (mg/portion) (QCT: 30mg/day)
n	tr	tr	0.5	0.3	0.1	0	6	1	17
0.1	tr	tr	0.3	0.3	0.1	0	5	0	11
n	tr	tr	0.2	0.2	0.1	0	2	n	13
n	0.1	0.1	1.1	0.2	0.2	0	17	2	27
0.4	tr	tr	0.5	0.3	tr	0	8	1	14
0.5	tr	0.1	0.8	0.2	0.1	0	33	2	32
0.1	tr	0.1	0.3	0.1	0.1	0	n	**3**	40
0.2	tr	tr	0.8	0.4	0.1	0	24	1	92
n	tr	**0.2**	**3.6**	0.7	0.2	0	14	n	tr
n	0.1	0.1	3.3	**0.8**	0.2	0	13	n	tr
n	0.1	0.1	1.3	0.5	0.3	0	9	n	1
tr	n	n	n	n	n	0	tr	n	tr
0.7	n	n	n	n	n	0	tr	n	tr
n	0.1	**0.2**	2.0	0.5	0.2	0	4	tr	tr
n	0.1	0.1	0.8	0.2	0.3	0	19	**3**	1

NUTS AND SEEDS

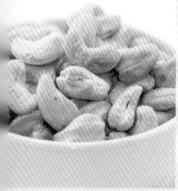

FOOD	AVERAGE PORTION SIZE	TOTAL CALORIES	FAT-SOLUBLE VITAMINS			
			A		D	
	grams per portion	kcals per portion	either Retinol (µg/portion) (QCT: 550µg/day)	or Carotene (µg/portion) (QCT: 3,300µg/day)	Cholecalciferol (µg/portion) (QCT: 0µg/day*)	*(*see pages 98–9)*
Almonds	50	**306**	0	0	0	
Brazil nuts	50	**341**	0	0	0	
Cashew nuts	50	**287**	0	0	0	
Chestnuts, dried	50	**160**	0	0	0	
Coconut, fresh	100	**351**	0	0	0	
Coconut, desiccated	50	**302**	0	0	0	
Hazelnuts	50	**325**	0	0	0	
Macadamia nuts (salted)	50	**374**	0	0	0	
Melon seeds	50	**292**	0	0	0	
Peanuts	50	**282**	0	0	0	
Peanut butter	20	**125**	0	0	0	
Pecan nuts	50	**345**	0	25	0	
Pine nuts	50	**344**	0	5	0	
Pistachio nuts (salted)	50	**301**	0	65	0	
Pumpkin seeds	50	**285**	0	**115**	0	
Sesame seeds	50	**299**	0	3	0	
Sesame spread (tahini)	50	**304**	0	0	0	
Sunflower seeds	50	**291**	0	7	0	
Walnuts	50	**344**	0	0	0	

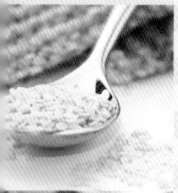

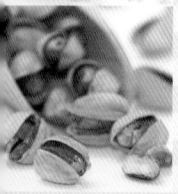

	WATER-SOLUBLE VITAMINS								
E	THE B-GROUP								C
Tocopherol (mg/portion) (QCT: 4mg/day)	Thiamin B1 (mg/portion) (QCT: 0.8mg/day)	Riboflavin B2 (mg/portion) (QCT: 1mg/day)	Niacin B3 (mg/portion) (QCT: 14mg/day)	Pantothenate B5 (mg/portion) (QCT: 5mg/day)	Pyridoxine B6 (mg/portion) (QCT: 1.3mg/day)	Cobalamin B12 (µg/portion) (QCT: 1µg/day)	Folate (µg/portion) (QCT: 150µg/day)	Biotin (µg/portion) (QCT: 30µg/day)	Ascorbic acid (mg/portion) (QCT: 30mg/day)
12.0	0.1	**0.4**	3.3	0.2	0.1	0	24	32	0
3.6	0.3	0	1.7	0.2	0.2	0	24	6	0
0.4	0.3	0.1	2.9	0.5	0.2	0	34	6	0
1.2	0.1	0	0.9	0.5	0.3	0	n	1	0
0.7	0	0	1.1	0.3	0.1	0	26	n	**3**
0.6	0	0	1.0	0.3	0	0	5	n	0
12.5	0.2	0.1	2.6	0.8	0.3	0	36	**38**	0
0.7	0.1	0	1.7	0.3	0.1	0	n	3	0
n	0.1	0.1	5.9	n	n	0	29	n	0
5.0	0.6	0.1	**9.7**	**1.3**	0.3	0	**55**	36	0
1.0	0	0	3.5	0.3	0.1	0	11	19	0
2.2	0.4	0.1	2.8	0.9	0.1	0	20	n	0
6.8	0.4	0.1	3.5	n	n	0	n	n	0
2.1	0.4	0.1	2.8	n	n	0	29	n	0
n	0.1	0.2	4.4	n	n	0	n	n	0
1.3	0.5	0.1	5.2	1.1	**0.4**	0	49	6	0
1.3	0.5	0.1	4.6	1.1	**0.4**	0	50	6	0
18.9	**0.8**	0.1	4.6	n	n	0	n	n	0
1.9	0.2	0.1	2.0	0.8	0.3	0	33	10	0

VEGETABLES AND PULSES

FOOD	AVERAGE PORTION SIZE	TOTAL CALORIES	FAT-SOLUBLE VITAMINS			
			A		D	
	grams per portion	kcals per portion	either Retinol (µg/portion) (QCT: 550µg/day)	or Carotene (µg/portion) (QCT: 3,300µg/day)	Cholecalciferol (µg/portion) (QCT: 0µg/day*)	(*see pages 98–9)
Root vegetables						
Beetroot	100	**36**	0	27	0	
Carrot	100	**35**	0	**8,115**	0	
Celeriac	100	**18**	0	26	0	
Parsnip	100	**64**	0	30	0	
Potato, baked	180	**245**	0	tr	0	
Potato, boiled in salted water	180	**130**	0	tr	0	
Potato, mashed	180	**187**	**74**	68	**0.7**	
Potato, chips (all types, average)	180	**398**	0	tr	0	
Swede	100	**24**	0	350	0	
Sweet potato, baked	130	**150**	0	6,682	0	
Beans, peas and lentils						
Aduki beans, cooked	100	**123**	0	6	0	
Baked beans, in tomato sauce	130	**105**	0	91	0	
Bean sprouts, fresh	60	**19**	0	24	0	
Black gram, blackeye, mung (av.)	100	**99**	0	12	0	
Broad beans, fresh	120	**71**	0	204	0	
Butter beans, cooked	100	**103**	0	tr	0	
Chick peas, cooked	100	**121**	0	23	0	
Green beans, fresh	100	**24**	0	330	0	
Haricot beans, cooked	100	**95**	0	tr	0	
Lentils, cooked (all types, av.)	100	**105**	0	20	0	
Peas, fresh	100	**83**	0	300	0	
Pinto beans, cooked	100	**137**	0	tr	0	
Red kidney beans, cooked	100	**103**	0	tr	0	
Runner beans, fresh	100	**22**	0	145	0	
Soya beans, cooked	100	**141**	0	tr	0	
Tempeh (fermented soya bean)	100	**166**	0	tr	0	
Tofu (soya bean curd)	100	**73**	0	tr	0	

continues

	WATER-SOLUBLE VITAMINS								
E	THE B-GROUP								C
Tocopherol (mg/portion) (QCT: 4mg/day)	Thiamin B1 (mg/portion) (QCT: 0.8mg/day)	Riboflavin B2 (mg/portion) (QCT: 1mg/day)	Niacin B3 (mg/portion) (QCT: 14mg/day)	Pantothenate B5 (mg/portion) (QCT: 5mg/day)	Pyridoxine B6 (mg/portion) (QCT: 1.3mg/day)	Cobalamin B12 (µg/portion) (QCT: 1µg/day)	Folate (µg/portion) (QCT: 150µg/day)	Biotin (µg/portion) (QCT: 30µg/day)	Ascorbic acid (mg/portion) (QCT: 30mg/day)
tr	tr	tr	0.4	0.1	tr	0	150	tr	5
0.6	0.1	tr	0.3	0.3	0.1	0	12	1	6
n	0.2	tr	0.4	n	0.1	0	51	n	14
1.0	0.2	tr	1.5	0.5	0.1	0	87	0	17
0.2	**0.7**	tr	3.6	0.8	1.0	0	79	1	25
0.1	0.3	tr	1.6	0.7	0.6	0	47	1	11
0.8	0.3	tr	1.6	0.6	0.5	tr	43	1	9
1.3	0.2	0.1	2.9	n	0.6	0	38	n	16
tr	0.2	tr	1.3	0.1	0.2	0	31	0	31
7.7	0.1	tr	1.0	0.8	0.1	0	n	0	30
n	0.1	0.1	2.4	n	n	0	n	n	tr
0.5	0.1	0.1	1.7	0.2	0.2	0	43	3	tr
0.1	0.1	tr	0.6	0.2	0.1	0	37	n	4
0.4	0.2	0.1	1.9	0.4	0.1	0	93	7	tr
0.6	tr	tr	**4.9**	**5.9**	0.1	0	174	3	38
0.4	0.2	0.1	1.5	0.4	0.2	0	n	n	tr
1.1	0.1	0.1	1.8	0.3	0.1	0	54	n	tr
0.2	0.1	0.1	1.4	0.1	0.1	0	80	1	12
0.1	0.1	tr	1.7	0.2	0.1	0	n	n	tr
n	0.1	0.1	1.8	0.3	0.3	0	30	n	tr
0.2	**0.7**	tr	3.6	0.2	0.1	0	62	1	24
n	0.2	0.1	1.7	0.3	0.2	0	145	n	2
0.2	0.2	0.1	1.9	0.2	0.1	0	42	n	1
0.2	0.1	tr	0.8	0.1	0.1	0	60	1	18
1.1	0.1	0.1	2.7	0.2	0.2	0	54	25	tr
1.0	0.1	tr	1.4	1.1	**1.9**	**1.0**	76	**53**	0
1.0	0.1	tr	1.4	4.9	0.1	0	15	n	0

VEGETABLES AND PULSES

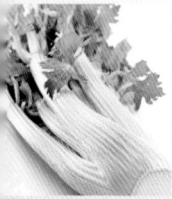

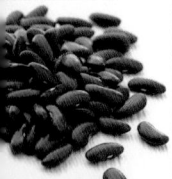

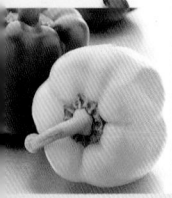

FOOD	AVERAGE PORTION SIZE	TOTAL CALORIES	FAT-SOLUBLE VITAMINS			
			A		D	
(where appropriate, numbers in brackets represent number of vegetables in average portion)	grams per portion	kcals per portion	either Retinol (µg/portion) (QCT: 550µg/day)	or Carotene (µg/portion) (QCT: 3,300µg/day)	Cholecalciferol (µg/portion) (QCT: 0µg/day*)	*(*see pages 98–9)*
Miscellaneous vegetables						
Artichoke hearts (2)	100	**18**	0	90	0	
Asparagus (5 spears)	125	**31**	0	394	0	
Aubergine (1/2)	130	**20**	0	91	0	
Avocado (1)	145	**276**	0	23	0	
Broccoli, green/purple	100	**34**	0	630	0	
Brussels sprouts (9)	100	**42**	0	215	0	
Cabbage (all types, average)	100	**26**	0	385	0	
Cauliflower	100	**34**	0	tr	0	
Celery (3 sticks)	100	**7**	0	50	0	
Courgette	100	**18**	0	610	0	
Cucumber (5 cm chunk)	120	**12**	0	192	0	
Curly kale	100	**33**	0	3,145	0	
Endive	100	**13**	0	440	0	
Fennel	100	**12**	0	140	0	
Lettuce (all types, average)	80	**10**	0	728	0	
Mushrooms, common	100	**13**	0	0	0	
Mushrooms, shiitake	50	**28**	0	0	0	
Okra	100	**31**	0	515	0	
Olive (10)	30	**31**	0	tr	0	
Onion/leek (all types, average)	100	**28**	0	350	0	
Pepper, green/red (1/2)**	80	**19**	0	212	0	
Pumpkin	180	**23**	0	1,719	0	
Seaweed, dried (all types, av.)***	10	**8**	0	527	0	
Spinach	100	**25**	0	3,535	0	
Spring greens	100	**33**	0	2,630	0	
Sweetcorn	100	**93**	0	97	0	
Swiss chard	100	**19**	0	4,625	0	
Tomato (1)	85	**14**	0	544	0	
Watercress	80	**18**	0	2,016	0	

***the carotene amount given is for green pepper – red pepper contains 3,070µg*
****nori contains the highest level of vitamin B12*

	WATER-SOLUBLE VITAMINS								
E	THE B-GROUP								C
Tocopherol (mg/portion) (QCT: 4mg/day)	Thiamin B1 (mg/portion) (QCT: 0.8mg/day)	Riboflavin B2 (mg/portion) (QCT: 1mg/day)	Niacin B3 (mg/portion) (QCT: 14mg/day)	Pantothenate B5 (mg/portion) (QCT: 5mg/day)	Pyridoxine B6 (mg/portion) (QCT: 1.3mg/day)	Cobalamin B12 (µg/portion) (QCT: 1µg/day)	Folate (µg/portion) (QCT: 150µg/day)	Biotin (µg/portion) (QCT: 30µg/day)	Ascorbic acid (mg/portion) (QCT: 30mg/day)
0.2	0.1	0.1	1.8	0.3	tr	0	68	4	2
1.5	0.2	0.1	1.9	0.2	0.1	0	**219**	1	15
tr	tr	tr	0.4	0.1	0.1	0	23	n	5
4.6	0.1	**0.3**	2.0	1.6	0.5	0	16	5	9
1.3	0.1	0.1	1.3	1.0	0.2	0	143	1	100
1.0	0.2	0.1	0.9	1.0	0.4	0	135	0	115
0.5	0.2	tr	0.8	0.2	0.2	0	75	tr	49
0.2	0.2	0.1	1.5	0.6	0.3	0	66	2	43
0.2	0.1	tr	0.4	0.4	tr	0	16	tr	8
n	0.1	tr	0.6	0.1	0.2	0	52	n	21
0.1	tr	tr	0.4	0.4	tr	0	11	1	2
1.7	0.1	0.1	1.7	0.1	0.3	0	120	1	110
n	0.1	0.1	0.6	0.9	tr	0	140	1	12
n	0.1	tr	0.6	n	0.1	0	42	n	5
0.5	0.1	tr	0.5	0.1	0.1	0	46	1	6
0.1	0.1	**0.3**	3.5	2.0	0.2	0	44	12	1
n	tr	0.1	0.8	n	n	n	n	n	tr
n	0.2	0.1	1.4	0.3	0.2	0	88	n	21
0.6	tr	tr	tr	tr	tr	0	tr	tr	0
0.6	0.2	0.1	0.8	0.1	0.4	0	40	1	11
0.6	0.0	tr	0.6	0.1	0.3	0	22	n	104
1.9	0.3	tr	0.4	0.7	tr	0	18	1	25
n	tr	0.1	0.4	n	tr	**1.0**	n	n	1
1.7	0.1	0.1	1.9	0.3	0.2	0	150	tr	26
n	0.1	0.1	2.0	0.4	0.2	0	92	0	**180**
0.7	0.2	0.1	2.3	0.7	0.2	0	41	n	8
n	tr	0.1	0.7	0.2	n	0	165	n	30
1.0	0.1	tr	0.9	0.2	0.1	0	14	1	14
1.2	0.1	tr	0.6	0.1	0.2	0	n	0	50

VEGETABLE DISHES

FOOD	AVERAGE PORTION SIZE	TOTAL CALORIES	FAT-SOLUBLE VITAMINS			
			A		D	
(where appropriate, numbers in brackets represent number of items in average portion)	grams per portion	kcals per portion	either Retinol (µg/portion) (QCT: 550µg/day)	or Carotene (µg/portion) (QCT: 3,300µg/day)	Cholecalciferol (µg/portion) (QCT: 0µg/day*)	*(*see pages 98–9)*
Bakes and flans						
Cannelloni	200	**290**	112	986	n	
Casserole, bean and vegetable	250	**115**	0	2,928	0	
Cauliflower cheese	200	**210**	140	145	0.5	
Flan, vegetable	120	**253**	92	2,606	0.7	
Lasagne, vegetable	450	**527**	n	n	n	
Moussaka, vegetable	350	**480**	n	n	n	
Nut roast	150	**528**	0	26	0	
Pizza, cheese and tomato	300	**711**	**177**	369	**5.4**	
Shepherd's pie, vegetable	300	**339**	87	1,755	tr	
Burgers, cutlets and pancakes						
Beanburger (no bun)	75	**152**	0	143	0	
Dosa with vegetable filling (1)	200	**307**	0	530	0	
Falafel (3)	100	**179**	0	230	0	
Nut cutlet (2)	120	**347**	0	624	0	
Onion bhaji/pakora (1)	50	**156**	0	55	0	
Pancake with vegetable filling (1)	200	**298**	132	300	1.4	
Quorn (myco-protein)	100	**86**	0	0	0	
Samosa, vegetable (1)	100	**217**	0	n	0	
Tempeh burger (1)	60	**116**	0	5	0	
Tofu burger (1)	60	**71**	0	396	0	
Vegeburger (1)	60	**147**	n	tr	n	
Curries, stews and rice dishes						
Bhaji, cauliflower	250	**535**	0	463	0	
Bhaji, mushroom	250	**415**	0	263	0	
Bhaji, potato	250	**395**	0	50	0	
Broccoli in cheese sauce	200	**236**	160	690	0.6	
Bubble and squeak	200	**248**	0	822	0	
Curry, cauliflower and potato	250	**148**	0	245	0	
Curry, chick pea and spinach	250	**498**	0	2,438	0	

continues

	WATER-SOLUBLE VITAMINS								
E	THE B-GROUP								C
Tocopherol (mg/portion) (QCT: 4mg/day)	Thiamin B1 (mg/portion) (QCT: 0.8mg/day)	Riboflavin B2 (mg/portion) (QCT: 1mg/day)	Niacin B3 (mg/portion) (QCT: 14mg/day)	Pantothenate B5 (mg/portion) (QCT: 5mg/day)	Pyridoxine B6 (mg/portion) (QCT: 1.3mg/day)	Cobalamin B12 (µg/portion) (QCT: 1µg/day)	Folate (µg/portion) (QCT: 150µg/day)	Biotin (µg/portion) (QCT: 30µg/day)	Ascorbic acid (mg/portion) (QCT: 30mg/day)
0.5	0.2	0.3	2.8	0.3	0.1	0.8	8	1	6
1.6	0.3	0.2	3.8	0.5	0.4	0	44	1	14
2.5	0.3	0.3	4.5	1.1	0.5	0.8	63	5	38
3.1	0.1	0.1	2.2	n	0.1	0.4	23	n	10
n	1.1	1.3	14.0	n	**2.0**	n	27	n	n
n	0.2	**2.5**	7.0	n	0.6	tr	42	n	n
8.3	0.7	0.5	**14.4**	1.3	0.4	tr	72	**35**	0
7.6	0.5	0.4	12.3	0.6	0.1	**3.0**	21	12	3
2.3	0.3	tr	2.4	0.7	0.5	tr	30	2	12
0.2	0.2	0.1	0.2	0.1	0.1	0	17	14	3
4.0	0.2	0.1	3.9	0.5	0.4	0	33	2	6
3.2	0.1	0.1	1.7	0.5	0.2	0	26	n	8
2.3	0.2	0.1	0.2	0.1	n	0	0	0	0
2.2	0.1	0.1	1.3	0.4	0.1	0	20	0	0
1.2	0.2	0.2	3.4	0.9	0.2	0.6	22	7	6
0	**3.7**	0.2	0.3	0.1	tr	0	7	9	0
n	0.1	0.1	0.2	n	0.2	0	44	n	n
0.9	0.1	0.1	1.1	n	n	0	8	n	tr
1.1	0.1	tr	1.0	0.2	0.1	0	10	n	1
n	1.3	0.2	3.7	n	0.2	n	49	n	n
12.4	0.4	0.1	4.0	1.3	0.6	0	88	3	**60**
10.0	0.3	0.4	5.0	**2.3**	0.4	0	40	14	5
6.1	0.4	0.1	2.5	0.7	0.9	0	43	1	18
2.0	0.1	0.3	3.8	n	0.2	0.6	86	n	54
n	0.2	tr	1.4	0.5	0.3	0	24	0	1
1.7	0.4	0.1	3.5	1.1	0.7	0	75	3	2
10.4	0.2	0.2	3.8	0.9	0.3	0	83	n	5

VEGETABLE DISHES

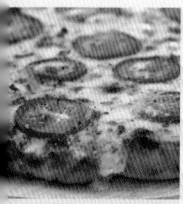

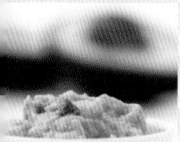

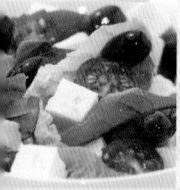

FOOD	AVERAGE PORTION SIZE	TOTAL CALORIES	FAT-SOLUBLE VITAMINS			
			A		D	
(where appropriate, numbers in brackets represent number of items in average portion)	grams per portion	kcals per portion	either Retinol (µg/portion) (QCT: 550µg/day)	or Carotene (µg/portion) (QCT: 3,300µg/day)	Cholecalciferol (µg/portion) (QCT: 0µg/day*)	*(*see pages 98–9)*
Curry, red lentil and mung bean	250	**285**	0	190	0	
Curry, red lentil and tomato	250	**230**	0	988	0	
Curry, okra	250	**273**	0	1,225	0	
Curry, mixed vegetable	250	**123**	0	2,313	0	
Okra with tomato and onion	250	**450**	0	1,588	0	
Ratatouille	250	**205**	0	463	0	
Risotto (brown rice)	350	**501**	0	1,803	0	
Side dishes, dips, spreads and sauces						
Guacamole	100	**128**	0	190	0	
Houmous	60	**112**	0	n	0	
Laverbread	100	**52**	0	n	0	
Pesto sauce	25	**129**	38	163	0	
Red cabbage, stewed with apple	100	**59**	0	37	0	
Tofu spread	50	**104**	0	135	0	
Vegetable pâté	50	**87**	tr	n	tr	
Vegetable stir-fry	100	**64**	0	n	0	
Vine leaves, stuffed with rice (3)	100	**262**	0	420	0	
Salads						
Coleslaw, with vinaigrette	100	**87**	0	735	0	
Salad, bean, with vinaigrette	100	**147**	0	250	0	
Salad, beetroot, with vinaigrette	100	**100**	0	22	0	
Salad, carrot, nut, with vinaigrette	100	**218**	0	**5,165**	0	
Salad, Greek	100	**130**	30	260	0.1	
Salad, green (no dressing)	100	**12**	0	195	0	
Salad, pasta, veg., w. mayonnaise	100	**127**	7	1,365	tr	
Salad, potato, with vinaigrette	100	**157**	0	50	0	
Salad, potato, with mayonnaise	100	**239**	23	70	0.1	
Salad, Waldorf	100	**193**	15	34	0.1	
Tabouleh orientale	100	**119**	0	260	0	

	WATER-SOLUBLE VITAMINS								
E	THE B-GROUP								C
Tocopherol (mg/portion) (QCT: 4mg/day)	Thiamin B1 (mg/portion) (QCT: 0.8mg/day)	Riboflavin B2 (mg/portion) (QCT: 1mg/day)	Niacin B3 (mg/portion) (QCT: 14mg/day)	Pantothenate B5 (mg/portion) (QCT: 5mg/day)	Pyridoxine B6 (mg/portion) (QCT: 1.3mg/day)	Cobalamin B12 (µg/portion) (QCT: 1µg/day)	Folate (µg/portion) (QCT: 150µg/day)	Biotin (µg/portion) (QCT: 30µg/day)	Ascorbic acid (mg/portion) (QCT: 30mg/day)
3.9	0.2	0.1	2.8	0.6	0.2	0	20	n	tr
4.7	0.2	0.1	2.5	0.5	0.3	0	13	n	13
n	0.4	0.1	3.3	0.5	0.5	0	80	n	23
2.0	0.2	0.1	1.8	0.4	0.3	0	38	2	18
n	0.5	0.1	3.5	0.6	0.5	0	**105**	n	30
6.7	0.2	0.1	2.0	n	0.4	0	103	n	35
4.4	0.6	0.3	8.1	1.5	0.4	0	42	n	35
2.4	0.1	0.1	1.2	0.8	0.3	0	12	3	11
n	0.1	tr	1.3	n	n	0	n	n	1
1.1	tr	0.1	1.1	n	n	tr	47	n	5
0.9	tr	0.1	1.4	n	n	0.2	n	n	1
0.2	tr	tr	0.5	0.2	0.1	0	14	0	21
2.5	tr	tr	0.4	tr	tr	0	7	n	2
n	1.1	0.7	3.2	n	0.2	tr	55	n	tr
n	0.1	0.1	1.3	n	0.3	0	16	n	8
1.1	0.1	0.1	0.9	0.1	0.1	0	6	1	4
0.9	0.1	tr	0.5	0.2	0.1	0	24	tr	24
0.5	0.1	tr	1.3	0.1	0.1	0	44	n	6
tr	tr	tr	0.5	0.1	0.1	0	86	tr	5
3.0	0.1	tr	0.8	0.3	0.2	0	17	9	4
1.1	tr	tr	1.0	0.2	0.1	0.1	16	n	26
0.4	0.1	tr	0.3	0.2	0.1	0	29	n	36
2.0	tr	tr	0.9	n	0.1	tr	16	n	21
0.1	0.2	tr	0.7	0.3	0.3	0	23	tr	7
5.3	0.1	tr	0.8	n	0.2	0.1	21	n	6
3.8	0.1	tr	0.1	0.2	0.1	0.1	7	n	5
1.2	0.1	tr	0.4	n	n	0	17	n	13

MEAT AND MEAT DISHES

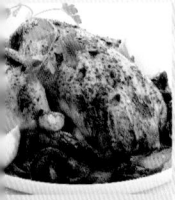

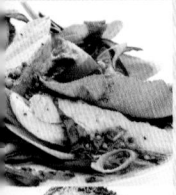

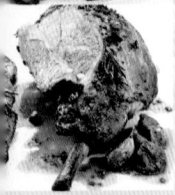

FOOD	AVERAGE PORTION SIZE	TOTAL CALORIES	FAT-SOLUBLE VITAMINS			
			A		D	
	grams per portion	kcals per portion	either Retinol (µg/portion) (QCT: 550µg/day)	or Carotene (µg/portion) (QCT: 3,300µg/day)	Cholecalciferol (µg/portion) (QCT: 0µg/day*)	(*see pages 98–9)
Beef						
Mince	200	**458**	tr	tr	tr	
Roast	120	**341**	tr	tr	tr	
Steak	120	**295**	tr	tr	tr	
Veal cutlet	150	**323**	tr	tr	tr	
Lamb						
Chop	160	**443**	tr	tr	tr	
Cutlet	100	**244**	tr	tr	tr	
Roast	120	**319**	tr	tr	tr	
Pork						
Bacon	100	**477**	tr	tr	tr	
Chop	120	**395**	tr	tr	tr	
Roast	120	**343**	tr	tr	tr	
Poultry and game						
Chicken, roast	120	**259**	tr	tr	tr	
Duck, roast	120	**407**	n	n	n	
Goose, roast	120	**383**	n	n	n	
Grouse, roast	120	**208**	n	n	n	
Hare/rabbit, roast or stewed	120	**230**	n	n	n	
Partridge, roast	120	**254**	n	n	n	
Pheasant, roast	120	**256**	n	n	n	
Pigeon, roast	120	**276**	n	n	n	
Turkey, roast	120	**205**	tr	tr	tr	
Venison, roast or stewed	120	**238**	n	n	n	
Offal						
Heart (all types, average)	100	**208**	tr	tr	n	
Kidney (all types, average)	100	**160**	123	n	n	
Liver (all types, average)	100	**213**	**13,540**	340	0.6	
Oxtail	100	**243**	tr	tr	tr	
Tripe	150	**150**	tr	tr	tr	

continues

	WATER-SOLUBLE VITAMINS								
E	THE B-GROUP								C
Tocopherol (mg/portion) (QCT: 4mg/day)	Thiamin B1 (mg/portion) (QCT: 0.8mg/day)	Riboflavin B2 (mg/portion) (QCT: 1mg/day)	Niacin B3 (mg/portion) (QCT: 14mg/day)	Pantothenate B5 (mg/portion) (QCT: 5mg/day)	Pyridoxine B6 (mg/portion) (QCT: 1.3mg/day)	Cobalamin B12 (µg/portion) (QCT: 1µg/day)	Folate (µg/portion) (QCT: 150µg/day)	Biotin (µg/portion) (QCT: 30µg/day)	Ascorbic acid (mg/portion) (QCT: 30mg/day)
0.6	0.1	0.7	18.6	1.6	0.6	4.0	32	tr	0
0.4	0.1	0.3	11.8	0.8	0.3	2.0	17	tr	0
0.4	tr	0.4	13.4	1.0	0.4	2.0	19	tr	0
n	n	n	10.1	n	n	2.0	tr	tr	0
0.1	0.1	0.3	12.6	0.6	0.2	3.0	3	2	0
0.1	0.1	0.1	6.4	0.4	0.2	1.0	3	1	0
0.1	0.1	0.4	13.2	0.7	0.2	2.0	4	1	0
0.2	0.4	0.2	9.5	0.3	0.3	tr	1	2	0
tr	0.7	0.2	8.6	0.8	0.3	2.0	4	2	0
tr	**0.8**	0.3	12.0	1.2	0.4	1.0	tr	2	0
0.1	0.1	0.2	15.4	1.4	0.3	tr	12	4	0
tr	0.3	0.6	12.6	1.4	0.3	4.0	12	2	0
n	n	n	6.6	n	0.5	n	n	n	n
n	0.4	0.6	17.5	n	n	n	n	n	n
0.2	0.1	0.3	16.3	1.0	0.6	14.0	5	1	0
n	n	n	8.3	n	n	n	n	n	n
n	tr	0.2	14.5	n	n	n	n	n	0
tr	n	n	16.9	n	n	n	n	n	0
tr	0.1	0.3	16.7	1.0	0.4	2.0	18	2	0
n	0.3	n	7.8	n	n	n	n	n	n
0.4	0.5	0.9	10.5	2.5	0.3	10.0	3	3	7
0.3	0.4	1.9	10.8	3.1	0.3	33.0	50	31	10
0.3	0.3	**3.1**	16.8	7.5	0.6	**75.0**	**298**	**70**	**17**
0.3	tr	0.3	8.8	1.0	0.3	3.0	7	1	0
0.1	tr	0.1	4.8	0.3	tr	tr	2	3	5

MEAT AND MEAT DISHES

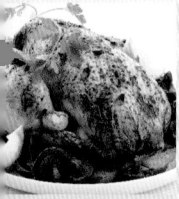

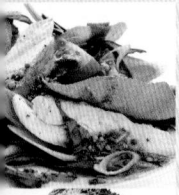

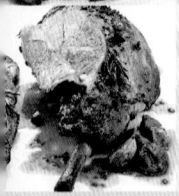

FOOD	AVERAGE PORTION SIZE	TOTAL CALORIES	FAT-SOLUBLE VITAMINS			
			A		D	
(where appropriate, numbers in brackets represent number of items in average portion)	grams per portion	kcals per portion	either Retinol (µg/portion) (QCT: 550µg/day)	or Carotene (µg/portion) (QCT: 3,300µg/day)	Cholecalciferol (µg/portion) (QCT: 0µg/day*)	*(*see pages 98–9)*
Cold meats						
Corned beef	25	**54**	tr	tr	tr	
Ham	25	**30**	tr	tr	tr	
Luncheon meat	25	**78**	tr	tr	tr	
Tongue	25	**53**	tr	tr	tr	
Burgers and sausages						
Beef burger, quarterpounder	80	**211**	tr	tr	tr	
Liver sausage (1)	50	**155**	4,150	tr	0.3	
Salami (2 slices)	34	**167**	tr	tr	tr	
Sausage (all types, average) (1)	50	**157**	tr	tr	tr	
Turkey burger/escalope	90	**119**	tr	tr	tr	
Meat dishes						
Black pudding	75	**229**	tr	tr	tr	
Bolognese sauce	220	**306**	tr	4,268	tr	
Chicken chow mein	350	**515**	tr	385	n	
Cornish pasty	155	**515**	tr	tr	tr	
Haggis	100	**310**	1,800	tr	0.1	
Hot pot	330	**376**	tr	**6,270**	tr	
Irish stew	330	**409**	tr	tr	tr	
Lamb curry	330	**528**	tr	tr	tr	
Lasagne	350	**669**	175	1,817	1.4	
Moussaka	330	**644**	99	215	0.2	
Pork pie	150	**564**	tr	tr	tr	
Samosa (lamb)	100	**578**	15	37	tr	
Sausage roll	60	**287**	75	tr	**0.7**	
Shepherd's pie/cottage pie	300	**357**	42	tr	0.4	
Shish kebab (in pitta with salad)	270	**419**	tr	324	0.5	
Spring roll	100	**242**	tr	175	n	
Steak and kidney pie	200	**646**	n	n	n	
Tandoori chicken	350	**749**	tr	735	**0.7**	

	WATER-SOLUBLE VITAMINS								
E	THE B-GROUP								C
Tocopherol (mg/portion) (QCT: 4mg/day)	Thiamin B1 (mg/portion) (QCT: 0.8mg/day)	Riboflavin B2 (mg/portion) (QCT: 1mg/day)	Niacin B3 (mg/portion) (QCT: 14mg/day)	Pantothenate B5 (mg/portion) (QCT: 5mg/day)	Pyridoxine B6 (mg/portion) (QCT: 1.3mg/day)	Cobalamin B12 (µg/portion) (QCT: 1µg/day)	Folate (µg/portion) (QCT: 150µg/day)	Biotin (µg/portion) (QCT: 30µg/day)	Ascorbic acid (mg/portion) (QCT: 30mg/day)
0.2	tr	0.1	2.3	0.1	tr	1.0	tr	1	0
tr	0.1	0.1	1.7	0.2	0.1	tr	tr	0	0
tr	tr	tr	1.1	0.1	tr	0	tr	tr	0
0.1	tr	0.1	1.6	0.1	tr	1.0	1	1	0
0.5	tr	0.2	6.4	0.4	0.2	2.0	12	2	0
0.1	0.1	0.8	3.8	0.8	0.1	4.0	10	4	tr
0.1	0.1	0.1	2.8	0.3	0.1	0	1	1	0
0.2	tr	0.1	2.7	0.3	0	1.0	tr	1	0
tr	0.1	0.1	14.0	0.6	0.3	1.0	12	1	0
0.2	0.1	0.1	2.9	0.5	tr	1.0	4	2	0
2.9	0.1	0.3	7.3	0.9	0.4	2.0	22	tr	11
3.4	0.2	0.1	10.9	1.6	0.3	tr	14	7	tr
2.0	0.2	0.1	5.1	0.9	0.2	2.0	5	2	0
0.4	0.2	0.4	3.5	0.5	0.1	2.0	8	12	tr
0.7	0.2	0.3	12.5	1.3	0.7	3.0	26	tr	**17**
0.4	0.2	0.2	10.2	1.0	0.5	3.0	20	3	13
2.7	0.1	0.3	9.6	1.0	0.3	3.0	17	3	7
2.8	0.4	0.4	12.6	1.4	0.5	4.0	25	7	7
1.1	0.2	0.5	11.2	1.7	0.6	3.0	26	7	13
0.6	0.2	0.1	5.9	0.9	0.1	2.0	5	2	0
n	0.1	0.1	2.7	n	n	tr	4	n	3
0.8	0.1	tr	2.0	0.1	tr	tr	2	1	0
0.8	0.1	0.4	9.6	0.9	0.5	3.0	21	tr	6
1.4	0.4	0.3	16.2	1.6	0.4	3.0	54	3	8
1.5	0.1	0.1	2.0	0.3	0.1	tr	3	3	tr
n	0.2	0.3	6.8	0.6	0.1	4.0	16	2	0
5.2	0.4	0.7	**56.0**	**7.9**	**2.1**	4.0	56	18	7

FISH AND FISH DISHES

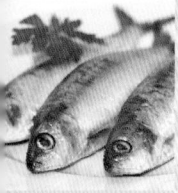

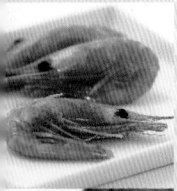

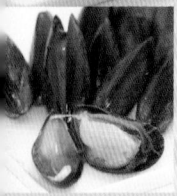

FOOD	AVERAGE PORTION SIZE	TOTAL CALORIES	FAT-SOLUBLE VITAMINS			
			A		D	
	grams per portion	kcals per portion	either Retinol (µg/portion) (QCT: 550µg/day)	or Carotene (µg/portion) (QCT: 3,300µg/day)	Cholecalciferol (µg/portion) (QCT: 0µg/day*)	(*see pages 98–9)
White fish						
Cod, fried in batter	120	**239**	n	tr	tr	
Cod, grilled	120	**114**	2	tr	tr	
Haddock, fried	120	**209**	tr	tr	tr	
Lemon sole, steamed	120	**109**	tr	tr	tr	
Plaice, fried in batter	120	**308**	n	tr	tr	
Skate, fried in batter	120	**202**	11	tr	n	
Oily fish						
Anchovies, canned	15	**29**	9	tr	n	
Herring, grilled	120	**217**	41	tr	19.3	
Kipper, grilled	120	**306**	46	tr	11.3	
Mackerel, smoked	150	**531**	47	tr	12.0	
Pilchards, in tomato sauce	50	**72**	4	70	7.0	
Salmon, canned	50	**77**	16	tr	4.6	
Salmon, grilled	100	**215**	16	tr	7.1	
Salmon, smoked	50	**71**	n	tr	n	
Sardines, canned	100	**172**	6	tr	4.6	
Trout, grilled	120	**162**	35	tr	11.5	
Tuna, canned	100	**99**	n	tr	3.6	
Seafood						
Lobster, boiled	90	**93**	tr	tr	tr	
Mussels, boiled	40	**42**	n	tr	tr	
Prawns, boiled	60	**59**	tr	tr	tr	
Shrimps, canned	50	**47**	tr	tr	tr	
Squid, fried in batter	65	**127**	30	tr	0.1	
Fish products and dishes						
Cod roe, fried	120	**242**	90	tr	**20.4**	
Fish fingers	60	**143**	tr	tr	tr	
Pasta with seafood	250	**275**	**130**	**130**	0	
Taramasalata	50	**252**	n	n	n	

	WATER-SOLUBLE VITAMINS								
E	THE B-GROUP								C
Tocopherol (mg/portion) (QCT: 4mg/day)	Thiamin B1 (mg/portion) (QCT: 0.8mg/day)	Riboflavin B2 (mg/portion) (QCT: 1mg/day)	Niacin B3 (mg/portion) (QCT: 14mg/day)	Pantothenate B5 (mg/portion) (QCT: 5mg/day)	Pyridoxine B6 (mg/portion) (QCT: 1.3mg/day)	Cobalamin B12 (µg/portion) (QCT: 1µg/day)	Folate (µg/portion) (QCT: 150µg/day)	Biotin (µg/portion) (QCT: 30µg/day)	Ascorbic acid (mg/portion) (QCT: 30mg/day)
n	0.1	0.1	4.4	0.4	0.2	2.4	**68**	4	tr
1.2	0.1	0.1	7.0	0.4	0.3	2.4	12	1	tr
n	0.1	0.1	6.6	0.3	0.3	1.2	n	2	tr
n	0.1	0.1	9.1	0.4	n	1.2	16	6	tr
n	0.2	0.4	5.5	1.0	0.1	n	32	**36**	tr
1.4	tr	0.1	6.1	n	n	n	n	n	tr
n	tr	tr	1.3	n	n	1.7	3	n	tr
0.8	tr	0.3	9.4	0.9	0.4	**18.0**	12	8	tr
0.4	tr	0.3	10.0	0.6	0.3	14.4	6	6	tr
0.4	0.4	**0.8**	**19.5**	1.6	**0.8**	9.0	n	5	tr
1.3	tr	0.2	4.5	0.4	0.1	6.5	n	6	tr
0.8	tr	0.1	5.2	0.4	0.1	2.0	7	5	tr
2.3	0.3	0.1	12.2	1.2	**0.8**	5.0	19	5	tr
n	0.1	0.1	6.8	0.4	0.1	1.5	1	n	tr
n	tr	0.3	10.1	0.8	0.2	13.0	8	10	tr
1.2	0.2	0.1	9.8	1.9	0.4	6.0	12	4	tr
0.6	tr	0.1	18.8	0.3	0.5	4.0	4	2	tr
1.3	0.1	0.1	5.0	0.9	0.1	2.7	8	6	tr
0.4	tr	0.2	2.0	0.2	tr	8.8	15	4	tr
n	tr	0.1	3.1	0.2	tr	4.8	n	1	tr
n	tr	tr	2.4	0.2	tr	1.0	8	1	tr
1.5	0.1	0.1	2.7	0.3	0.2	1.3	10	n	tr
n	**0.7**	0.4	5.9	**3.1**	0.3	13.2	n	18	tr
n	0.1	tr	2.5	0.2	0.1	0.6	10	1	tr
1.0	0.1	0.2	6.8	0.5	0.2	2.5	15	3	**3**
n	tr	0.1	0.5	n	n	1.5	2	n	1

DAIRY PRODUCTS

FOOD	AVERAGE PORTION SIZE	TOTAL CALORIES	FAT-SOLUBLE VITAMINS			
			A		D	
	grams/ml per portion	kcals per portion	either Retinol (µg/portion) (QCT: 550µg/day)	or Carotene (µg/portion) (QCT: 3,300µg/day)	Cholecalciferol (µg/portion) (QCT: 0µg/day*)	*(*see pages 98–9)*
Milk						
Skimmed milk	200	**64**	tr	tr	tr	
Semi-skimmed milk	200	**92**	38	tr	tr	
Whole milk	200	**132**	66	40	tr	
Goat's milk	200	**124**	88	tr	tr	
Soya milk, unsweetened	200	**52**	tr	tr	0	
Milkshake, thick	200	**176**	70	22	tr	
Cream						
Single cream	30	**58**	87	51	4.0	
Double cream	30	**149**	234	**145**	4.0	
Crème fraîche	30	**113**	116	43	4.0	
Cheeses						
Brie/camembert	40	**137**	119	77	3.0	
Cheddar	40	**166**	146	56	5.0	
Cottage cheese	40	**40**	18	tr	0	
Cream cheese	40	**176**	154	88	5.0	
Danish blue	40	**137**	98	113	3.0	
Edam	40	**136**	75	73	3.0	
Feta	40	**100**	88	tr	8.0	
Goats cheese, soft	40	**128**	133	tr	8.0	
Gouda	40	**151**	103	56	3.0	
Mozzarella, fresh	40	**103**	103	61	3.0	
Parmesan, fresh	40	**166**	148	93	5.0	
Stilton	40	**164**	144	73	3.0	
Yogurt						
Whole-milk yogurt, plain	150	**119**	42	32	0	
Greek-style yogurt, plain	150	**200**	173	tr	6.0	
Greek-style yogurt, sheep's milk	150	**138**	129	17	**12.0**	
Soya yogurt, with fruit	150	**110**	35	tr	0	
Fromage frais, plain	100	**113**	82	tr	0	

continues

	WATER-SOLUBLE VITAMINS								
E	THE B-GROUP								C
Tocopherol (mg/portion) (QCT: 4mg/day)	Thiamin B1 (mg/portion) (QCT: 0.8mg/day)	Riboflavin B2 (mg/portion) (QCT: 1mg/day)	Niacin B3 (mg/portion) (QCT: 14mg/day)	Pantothenate B5 (mg/portion) (QCT: 5mg/day)	Pyridoxine B6 (mg/portion) (QCT: 1.3mg/day)	Cobalamin B12 (µg/portion) (QCT: 1µg/day)	Folate (µg/portion) (QCT: 150µg/day)	Biotin (µg/portion) (QCT: 30µg/day)	Ascorbic acid (mg/portion) (QCT: 30mg/day)
tr	0.1	0.4	1.6	1.0	0.1	1.6	18	5	2
0.1	0.1	0.5	1.8	0.6	0.1	0.8	12	4	2
1.6	0.1	0.5	1.6	1.2	0.1	1.8	16	5	**4**
0.1	0.1	0.1	1.6	0.8	0.1	0.2	2	6	2
0.6	0.1	0.1	1.6	tr	0.1	0	28	2	0
0.2	0.1	0.5	1.6	0.6	0.1	1.0	8	4	2
0.1	tr	0.1	0.2	0.1	tr	0.1	2	1	tr
0.5	tr	0.1	0.1	0.1	tr	0.2	2	tr	tr
0.2	tr	0.1	tr	n	tr	0.1	1	n	n
0.3	tr	0.1	2.0	0.2	0.1	0.2	22	1	tr
0.2	tr	0.2	2.8	0.2	0.1	1.0	12	2	tr
0	tr	0.1	1.4	0.1	tr	0.2	9	2	tr
0.4	tr	0.1	0.3	0.1	tr	0.1	4	1	tr
0.3	tr	0.2	2.4	0.2	tr	0.5	22	1	tr
0.3	tr	0.1	2.5	0.2	tr	0.8	16	1	tr
0.1	tr	0.1	1.5	0.1	tr	0.4	9	1	tr
0.3	tr	0.2	2.7	0.2	tr	0.2	9	2	tr
0.2	tr	0.1	2.8	0.1	tr	0.7	17	1	tr
0.1	tr	0.2	2.0	0.1	tr	0.7	8	1	tr
0.3	tr	0.1	3.6	0.2	tr	1.3	5	1	tr
0.2	tr	0.2	2.6	0.4	0.1	0.5	31	1	tr
0.1	0.1	0.4	2.3	0.8	**0.2**	0.3	27	4	2
0.6	**0.2**	0.2	2.4	n	tr	0.3	9	n	tr
1.1	0.1	0.5	1.8	n	0.1	0.3	5	n	tr
2.9	**0.2**	tr	n	0.2	tr	0	n	2	0
0.2	0.1	0.2	1.3	0.5	tr	0.5	15	tr	tr

DAIRY PRODUCTS

FOOD	AVERAGE PORTION SIZE	TOTAL CALORIES	FAT-SOLUBLE VITAMINS			
			A		D	
	grams per portion	kcals per portion	either Retinol (µg/portion) (QCT: 550µg/day)	or Carotene (µg/portion) (QCT: 3,300µg/day)	Cholecalciferol (µg/portion) (QCT: 0µg/day*)	*(*see pages 98–9)*
Ice cream						
Dairy ice cream	100	**215**	164	80	**12.0**	
Non-dairy ice cream	100	**153**	tr	tr	tr	
Eggs and egg dishes						
Egg, boiled	50	**74**	95	tr	0.9	
Egg, fried	60	**107**	129	tr	0.5	
Egg, scrambled	120	**308**	**384**	125	0.8	
Omelette	120	**234**	296	64	0.8	
Quiche	120	**378**	221	71	0.4	

	WATER-SOLUBLE VITAMINS								
E	THE B-GROUP								C
Tocopherol (mg/portion) (QCT: 4mg/day)	Thiamin B1 (mg/portion) (QCT: 0.8mg/day)	Riboflavin B2 (mg/portion) (QCT: 1mg/day)	Niacin B3 (mg/portion) (QCT: 14mg/day)	Pantothenate B5 (mg/portion) (QCT: 5mg/day)	Pyridoxine B6 (mg/portion) (QCT: 1.3mg/day)	Cobalamin B12 (µg/portion) (QCT: 1µg/day)	Folate (µg/portion) (QCT: 150µg/day)	Biotin (µg/portion) (QCT: 30µg/day)	Ascorbic acid (mg/portion) (QCT: 30mg/day)
0.3	0.1	0.3	1.1	1.1	tr	0.5	6	2	1
0.6	0.1	0.3	0.9	0.4	tr	0	8	3	1
0.6	tr	0.2	1.9	0.7	tr	0.6	20	8	0
n	tr	0.2	3.1	0.8	0.1	1.0	24	11	0
1.5	0.1	0.4	3.8	**1.6**	0.1	**2.6**	**36**	20	tr
1.3	0.1	0.4	4.0	**1.6**	0.1	**2.6**	**36**	**21**	tr
2.7	0.1	0.3	**4.3**	0.7	0.1	1.8	19	9	1

FATS AND OILS

FOOD	AVERAGE PORTION SIZE	TOTAL CALORIES	FAT-SOLUBLE VITAMINS			
			A		D	
(amounts in brackets represent size of average portion)	grams/ml per portion	kcals per portion	either Retinol (µg/portion) (QCT: 550µg/day)	or Carotene (µg/portion) (QCT: 3,300µg/day)	Cholecalciferol (µg/portion) (QCT: 0µg/day*)	*(*see pages 98–9)*
Cooking fats (1 tbs)						
Ghee, butter	15	**135**	101	0	0.1	
Ghee, vegetable	15	**134**	tr	tr	0	
Lard	15	**134**	tr	tr	n	
Suet, beef	15	**124**	8	tr	tr	
Suet, vegetable	15	**125**	0	0	0	
Table fats (on 1 slice of bread)						
Butter	10	**74**	82	43	0.1	
Spread (eg. Clover)	10	**68**	57	45	0.4	
Low-fat spread (eg. Anchor)	10	**39**	16	43	tr	
Margarine, hard (eg. Stork)	10	**72**	67	**75**	0.8	
- hard veg. (eg. Tomor)	10	**74**	67	**75**	0.8	
- polyunsat. (eg. Blue Band)	10	**75**	68	35	0.8	
Spread (70–80% fat, eg. Flora)	10	**64**	n	n	n	
- (60% fat, eg. Vitalite Light)	10	**55**	98	tr	n	
- with olive oil (eg. Bertolli)	10	**57**	n	n	n	
- (35–40% fat, eg. Gold Sunfl.)	10	**37**	n	n	n	
- (20–25% fat, eg. Outline)	10	**25**	47	58	0.8	
Oils (1 tbs)						
Cod liver oil	15	**135**	**270**	tr	**31.5**	
Corn oil	15	**135**	0	tr	0	
Evening primrose oil	15	**135**	0	tr	0	
Grapeseed oil	15	**135**	0	tr	0	
Olive oil	15	**135**	0	tr	0	
Safflower oil	15	**135**	0	tr	0	
Sesame oil	15	**135**	0	tr	0	
Sunflower oil	15	**135**	0	tr	0	
Vegetable oil, blended	15	**135**	0	tr	0	
Walnut oil	15	**135**	0	tr	0	
Wheat germ oil	15	**135**	0	tr	0	

E	WATER-SOLUBLE VITAMINS								C
	THE B-GROUP								
Tocopherol (mg/portion) (QCT: 4mg/day)	Thiamin B1 (mg/portion) (QCT: 0.8mg/day)	Riboflavin B2 (mg/portion) (QCT: 1mg/day)	Niacin B3 (mg/portion) (QCT: 14mg/day)	Pantothenate B5 (mg/portion) (QCT: 5mg/day)	Pyridoxine B6 (mg/portion) (QCT: 1.3mg/day)	Cobalamin B12 (µg/portion) (QCT: 1µg/day)	Folate (µg/portion) (QCT: 150µg/day)	Biotin (µg/portion) (QCT: 30µg/day)	Ascorbic acid (mg/portion) (QCT: 30mg/day)
0.1	tr	tr	tr	tr	tr	tr	tr	tr	0
1.5	tr	tr	tr	tr	tr	tr	tr	tr	0
0.2	tr	tr	tr	tr	tr	tr	tr	tr	0
0.2	tr	tr	tr	tr	tr	tr	tr	tr	0
2.7	tr	tr	tr	tr	tr	tr	tr	tr	0
0.2	tr	tr	tr	tr	tr	tr	tr	tr	0
1.1	tr	tr	tr	tr	tr	tr	tr	tr	0
0.4	tr	tr	tr	tr	tr	tr	tr	tr	0
0.4	tr	tr	tr	tr	tr	tr	tr	tr	0
n	tr	tr	tr	tr	tr	tr	tr	tr	0
3.3	tr	tr	tr	tr	tr	tr	tr	tr	0
3.8	tr	tr	tr	tr	tr	tr	tr	tr	0
3.1	tr	tr	tr	tr	tr	tr	tr	tr	0
n	tr	tr	tr	tr	tr	tr	tr	tr	0
n	tr	tr	tr	tr	tr	tr	tr	tr	0
0.5	tr	tr	tr	tr	tr	tr	tr	tr	0
3.0	tr	tr	tr	tr	tr	tr	tr	tr	0
2.6	tr	tr	tr	tr	tr	tr	tr	tr	0
n	tr	tr	tr	tr	tr	tr	tr	tr	0
n	tr	tr	tr	tr	tr	tr	tr	tr	0
0.8	tr	tr	tr	tr	tr	tr	tr	tr	0
6.1	tr	tr	tr	tr	tr	tr	tr	tr	0
n	tr	tr	tr	tr	tr	tr	tr	tr	0
7.4	tr	tr	tr	tr	tr	tr	tr	tr	0
n	tr	tr	tr	tr	tr	tr	tr	tr	0
n	tr	tr	tr	tr	tr	tr	tr	tr	0
20.5	tr	tr	tr	tr	tr	tr	tr	tr	0

GRAINS, CEREALS, BREADS

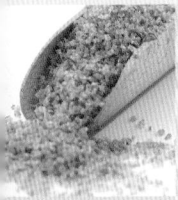

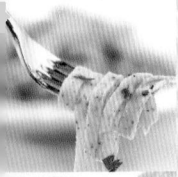

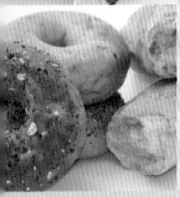

FOOD	AVERAGE PORTION SIZE	TOTAL CALORIES	FAT-SOLUBLE VITAMINS			
			A		D	
	grams per portion	kcals per portion	either Retinol (µg/portion) (QCT: 550µg/day)	or Carotene (µg/portion) (QCT: 3,300µg/day)	Cholecalciferol (µg/portion) (QCT: 0µg/day*)	(*see pages 98–9)
Flours and grains						
Barley, pearl	100	**360**	0	0	0	
Buckwheat	100	**364**	0	0	0	
Bulgur wheat	100	**353**	0	n	0	
Cornflour	100	**354**	0	0	0	
Couscous	100	**227**	0	tr	0	
Custard powder	100	**354**	0	0	0	
Millet	100	**354**	0	0	0	
Oatmeal	100	**401**	0	0	0	
Quinoa	100	**309**	0	n	0	
Rice, brown	200	**282**	0	0	0	
Rice, white	200	**276**	0	0	0	
Rice flour	100	**366**	0	0	0	
Rye flour	100	**335**	0	0	0	
Soya flour	100	**447**	0	n	0	
Wheat flour, white	100	**341**	0	0	0	
Wheat flour, wholemeal	100	**310**	0	0	0	
Wheat germ	25	**76**	0	0	0	
Wheat bran	15	**31**	0	3	0	
Noodles and pasta (cooked)						
Noodles, egg	300	**186**	6	0	0	
Noodles, plain	300	**186**	0	0	0	
Pasta, white	300	**312**	0	0	0	
Pasta, wholemeal	300	**339**	0	0	0	
Pastry						
Puff pastry	100	**373**	0	0	n	
Shortcrust pastry	100	**449**	120	0	1.2	
Breakfast cereals						
All-bran	50	**126**	0	11	1.4	
Coco pops	50	**193**	0	11	1.4	

continues

	WATER-SOLUBLE VITAMINS								
E	THE B-GROUP								C
Tocopherol (mg/portion) (QCT: 4mg/day)	Thiamin B1 (mg/portion) (QCT: 0.8mg/day)	Riboflavin B2 (mg/portion) (QCT: 1mg/day)	Niacin B3 (mg/portion) (QCT: 14mg/day)	Pantothenate B5 (mg/portion) (QCT: 5mg/day)	Pyridoxine B6 (mg/portion) (QCT: 1.3mg/day)	Cobalamin B12 (µg/portion) (QCT: 1µg/day)	Folate (µg/portion) (QCT: 150µg/day)	Biotin (µg/portion) (QCT: 30µg/day)	Ascorbic acid (mg/portion) (QCT: 30mg/day)
0.4	0.1	0.1	0.1	0.5	0.2	0	20	tr	0
tr	0.3	0.1	4.5	1.2	0.4	0	n	n	0
n	0.5	0.1	6.1	n	n	0	n	n	0
tr	tr	tr	tr	tr	tr	0	tr	tr	0
n	0.2	0.1	1.9	n	n	0	n	n	0
tr	tr	tr	tr	tr	tr	0	tr	tr	0
tr	0.7	0.2	2.8	n	n	0	n	n	0
1.5	0.9	0.1	3.4	1.2	0.3	0	60	**21**	0
n	0.2	0.4	4.8	n	n	0	n	n	0
0.6	0.3	tr	3.8	n	n	0	20	n	0
tr	tr	tr	3.0	tr	0.1	0	8	2	0
n	0.1	0.1	3.5	n	0.2	0	n	n	0
1.6	0.4	0.2	2.6	1.0	0.4	0	78	6	0
1.5	0.8	0.3	**10.6**	**1.6**	0.5	0	**345**	n	0
0.3	0.3	tr	3.6	0.3	0.2	0	22	1	0
1.4	0.5	0.1	8.3	0.1	0.5	0	57	7	0
5.5	0.5	0.2	2.5	0.5	0.8	0	83	6	0
0.4	0.1	0.1	4.9	0.4	0.2	0	39	7	0
n	tr	tr	2.1	n	tr	tr	3	n	0
tr	0.1	tr	2.4	tr	tr	0	6	tr	0
tr	tr	tr	3.6	tr	0.1	0	12	tr	0
tr	0.6	0.1	6.9	0.6	0.2	0	21	tr	0
n	0.2	tr	2.1	n	0.1	tr	16	n	0
1.4	0.2	tr	2.1	0.2	0.1	0	13	1	0
0.1	0.2	0.1	3.0	0.3	0.1	0	31	3	0
0.1	0.2	0.1	3.0	0.3	0.1	0	31	3	0

GRAINS, CEREALS, BREADS

FOOD	AVERAGE PORTION SIZE	TOTAL CALORIES	FAT-SOLUBLE VITAMINS			
			A		D	
(where appropriate, numbers in brackets represent number of items in average portion)	grams per portion	kcals per portion	either Retinol (µg/portion) (QCT: 550µg/day)	or Carotene (µg/portion) (QCT: 3,300µg/day)	Cholecalciferol (µg/portion) (QCT: 0µg/day*)	*(*see pages 98–9)*
Corn flakes	50	**178**	0	11	1.4	
Fruit 'n' Fibre	50	**176**	0	11	1.4	
Grapenuts	50	**173**	0	11	2.2	
Muesli (Swiss style)	70	**255**	0	15	0	
Porridge (made with water)	200	**98**	0	0	0	
Puffed wheat	50	**161**	0	11	0	
Rice Krispies	50	**185**	0	11	1.4	
Shredded wheat (2)	50	**163**	0	11	0	
Special K	50	**190**	0	11	1.4	
Weetabix (2)	40	**142**	0	8	0	
Breads and rolls						
Bagel (1)	90	**246**	0	**19**	**2.5**	
Brown bread (1 slice)	40	**87**	0	8	0	
Chapati (1)	55	**111**	0	12	0	
French baguette (5 cm slice)	40	**108**	0	8	0	
Granary bread (1 slice)	40	**94**	0	8	0	
Naan bread (1)	160	**538**	**155**	0	0.3	
Papadum (fried) (2)	26	**96**	0	n	0	
Pitta bread (1 large)	95	**252**	0	0	0	
Rye bread (1 slice)	25	**55**	0	0	0	
Wheat germ bread (1 slice)	40	**105**	0	8	0	
White bread (1 slice)	40	**94**	0	8	0	
Wholemeal bread (1 slice)	40	**86**	0	8	0	
Croissant (1)	50	**180**	11	11	0.1	
Hamburger bun (1)	50	**132**	n	0	n	
Morning roll (1)	50	**135**	0	11	0	
Wholemeal roll (1)	50	**121**	0	11	0	

	WATER-SOLUBLE VITAMINS								
E	THE B-GROUP								C
Tocopherol (mg/portion) (QCT: 4mg/day)	Thiamin B1 (mg/portion) (QCT: 0.8mg/day)	Riboflavin B2 (mg/portion) (QCT: 1mg/day)	Niacin B3 (mg/portion) (QCT: 14mg/day)	Pantothenate B5 (mg/portion) (QCT: 5mg/day)	Pyridoxine B6 (mg/portion) (QCT: 1.3mg/day)	Cobalamin B12 (µg/portion) (QCT: 1µg/day)	Folate (µg/portion) (QCT: 150µg/day)	Biotin (µg/portion) (QCT: 30µg/day)	Ascorbic acid (mg/portion) (QCT: 30mg/day)
0.1	0.2	0.1	0	0.3	0.1	0	31	3	0
0.1	0.2	0.1	3.0	0.3	0.1	0	31	3	0
0.1	0.2	0.1	3.0	0.3	0.1	0	31	3	0
0.1	0.2	0.1	4.1	0.4	0.1	0	43	4	0
0.4	**1.2**	tr	0.8	0.2	tr	0	8	4	0
1.0	tr	tr	4.1	0.3	0.1	0	10	4	0
0.3	0.5	0.8	8.7	0.4	0.9	1.0	125	1	0
0.6	0.1	tr	3.3	0.4	0.1	0	15	5	0
0.3	0.6	0.9	10.6	0.3	1.1	1.0	150	2	0
0.4	0.3	0.4	4.8	0.3	0.1	0	20	3	0
0.5	0.9	**1.4**	**15.7**	0.6	**1.6**	**2**	225	2	0
tr	0.1	tr	1.7	0.1	0.1	0	16	1	0
tr	0.1	tr	1.7	0.1	0.1	0	8	1	0
0.1	0.1	tr	2.4	0.2	0.1	0	16	2	0
n	0.1	tr	2.0	n	0.1	0	36	n	tr
2.2	0.3	0.2	4.8	0.5	0.1	tr	22	3	0
n	tr	tr	0.9	n	n	0	7	n	0
n	0.2	0.1	3.2	n	n	0	20	n	0
0.3	0.1	tr	1.0	0.1	tr	0	6	n	0
n	0.2	tr	2.0	0.1	0.1	0	18	1	0
tr	0.1	tr	1.4	0.1	tr	0	12	0	0
tr	0.1	tr	1.3	0.1	tr	0	10	0	0
tr	0.1	0.1	1.9	0.3	0.1	tr	37	5	0
tr	0.1	0.1	1.7	0.2	tr	tr	24	1	0
tr	0.1	tr	2.2	0.2	tr	0	16	1	0
0.1	0.2	0.1	3.0	0.3	0.1	0	31	3	0

BISCUITS, CAKES, PUDDINGS

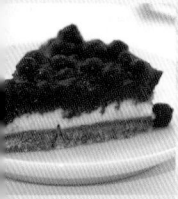

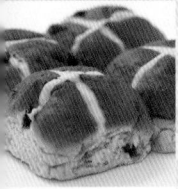

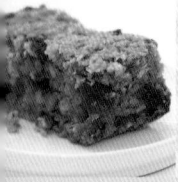

FOOD	AVERAGE PORTION SIZE	TOTAL CALORIES	FAT-SOLUBLE VITAMINS			
			A		D	
(where appropriate, numbers in brackets represent number of items in average portion)	grams per portion	kcals per portion	either Retinol (µg/portion) (QCT: 550µg/day)	or Carotene (µg/portion) (QCT: 3,300µg/day)	Cholecalciferol (µg/portion) (QCT: 0µg/day*)	*(*see pages 98–9)*
Biscuits						
Chocolate biscuit (1)	25	**131**	tr	5	0	
Cream cracker (1)	15	**66**	0	3	0	
Crispbread, rye (1)	10	**32**	0	2	0	
Digestive biscuit, plain (1)	15	**71**	0	3	0	
Flapjack (1)	60	**290**	138	13	1.4	
Wholemeal biscuit (1)	15	**54**	12	3	0.1	
Oatcake (1)	15	**66**	0	3	0	
Rich tea/Marie biscuit (1)	10	**46**	0	2	0	
Shortbread (1)	15	**75**	41	3	tr	
Water biscuit (1)	10	**44**	0	2	0	
Wholemeal cracker (1)	15	**62**	0	3	0	
Cakes						
Chocolate cake (1 slice)	70	**319**	189	15	1.7	
Fruit cake (1 slice)	70	**248**	n	15	n	
Gâteau (1 slice)	70	**236**	221	0	0.4	
Sponge cake (1 slice)	70	**321**	196	15	**1.8**	
Swiss roll (1 slice)	35	**97**	28	7	0.2	
Puddings						
Cheesecake (1 slice)	110	**452**	**385**	n	1.0	
Christmas pudding	100	**291**	25	n	0.1	
Fruit crumble	170	**337**	n	n	1.1	
Custard (made with milk)	150	**176**	96	n	tr	
Fruit pie	120	**223**	56	n	0.4	
Pancake (1)	110	**331**	64	n	0.2	
Rice pudding	200	**178**	n	n	n	
Trifle	170	**272**	128	n	0.2	
Buns and pastries						
Crumpet (1)	40	**71**	0	0	0	
Currant bun (1)	60	**178**	n	n	0	

continues

	WATER-SOLUBLE VITAMINS								
E	THE B-GROUP								C
Tocopherol (mg/portion) (QCT: 4mg/day)	Thiamin B1 (mg/portion) (QCT: 0.8mg/day)	Riboflavin B2 (mg/portion) (QCT: 1mg/day)	Niacin B3 (mg/portion) (QCT: 14mg/day)	Pantothenate B5 (mg/portion) (QCT: 5mg/day)	Pyridoxine B6 (mg/portion) (QCT: 1.3mg/day)	Cobalamin B12 (µg/portion) (QCT: 1µg/day)	Folate (µg/portion) (QCT: 150µg/day)	Biotin (µg/portion) (QCT: 30µg/day)	Ascorbic acid (mg/portion) (QCT: 30mg/day)
0.4	tr	tr	0.4	n	tr	0	n	n	0
0.2	tr	tr	0.5	tr	tr	0	3	tr	0
0.1	tr	tr	0.3	0.1	tr	0	4	1	0
n	tr	tr	0.4	n	tr	0	2	n	0
1.7	0.2	tr	0.8	0.2	0.1	0	7	5	0
0.3	0.1	tr	1.1	0.1	0.1	tr	4	1	0
0.3	0.1	tr	0.5	0.2	tr	0	4	3	0
0.1	tr	tr	0.3	n	tr	0	1	n	0
0.1	tr	tr	0.3	tr	tr	0	1	tr	0
n	tr	tr	0.3	n	tr	0	n	n	0
0.2	tr	tr	0.7	0.1	tr	0	4	1	0
1.9	0.1	0.1	1.8	0.4	tr	0.7	8	6	0
n	0.1	0.1	1.1	n	n	0	n	n	0
n	0.1	0.2	1.5	0.4	tr	0.9	9	7	0
2.0	0.1	0.1	1.8	0.4	tr	0.7	7	5	0
0.3	tr	0.1	0.8	0.2	tr	0.4	5	4	tr
n	tr	0.2	1.7	n	tr	tr	8	n	1
0.6	0.1	0.1	1.7	0.2	0.1	tr	8	4	0
1.7	0.1	tr	1.5	0.2	0.1	0	5	tr	5
0.2	0.1	**0.3**	1.5	0.6	0.1	**1.5**	9	3	2
0.8	0.1	tr	1.1	0.1	tr	0	4	tr	6
0.4	0.1	0.2	2.1	0.6	0.1	1.1	9	6	1
n	0.1	**0.3**	1.8	n	tr	tr	n	n	0
0.7	0.1	0.2	2.0	0.5	0.1	tr	15	5	**7**
0.1	0.1	tr	0.8	0.1	tr	tr	3	2	0
n	0.2	0.1	1.3	n	0.1	tr	24	n	0

BISCUITS, CAKES, PUDDINGS

FOOD	AVERAGE PORTION SIZE	TOTAL CALORIES	FAT-SOLUBLE VITAMINS			
			A		D	
(where appropriate, numbers in brackets represent number of items in average portion)	grams per portion	kcals per portion	either Retinol (µg/portion) (QCT: 550µg/day)	or Carotene (µg/portion) (QCT: 3,300µg/day)	Cholecalciferol (µg/portion) (QCT: 0µg/day*)	*(*see pages 98–9)*
Danish pastry (1)	110	**411**	n	n	n	
Doughnut (jam) (1)	75	**252**	n	n	n	
Greek pastry (Baklava) (1)	100	**322**	n	0	n	
Hot cross bun (1)	50	**155**	34	11	0.3	
Jam tart (1)	25	**95**	16	5	0.2	
Mince pie (1)	50	**212**	41	11	0.4	
Muffin (American) (1)	70	**256**	0	15	0	
Muffin (English) (1)	70	**198**	47	15	0.3	
Scone (1)	50	**181**	70	11	0.6	
Teacake (1)	60	**178**	n	13	0	
Waffle (1)	65	**217**	130	14	0.2	

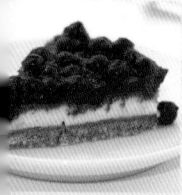

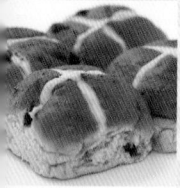

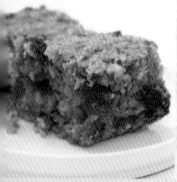

	WATER-SOLUBLE VITAMINS								
E	THE B-GROUP								C
Tocopherol (mg/portion) (QCT: 4mg/day)	Thiamin B1 (mg/portion) (QCT: 0.8mg/day)	Riboflavin B2 (mg/portion) (QCT: 1mg/day)	Niacin B3 (mg/portion) (QCT: 14mg/day)	Pantothenate B5 (mg/portion) (QCT: 5mg/day)	Pyridoxine B6 (mg/portion) (QCT: 1.3mg/day)	Cobalamin B12 (µg/portion) (QCT: 1µg/day)	Folate (µg/portion) (QCT: 150µg/day)	Biotin (µg/portion) (QCT: 30µg/day)	Ascorbic acid (mg/portion) (QCT: 30mg/day)
tr	0.1	0.1	2.3	0.6	0.1	tr	22	**8**	0
tr	0.2	0.1	1.9	n	0.1	tr	16	n	n
n	0.1	tr	2.0	n	n	n	n	n	n
0.4	0.1	0.1	1.4	0.2	0.1	tr	14	3	0
0.2	tr	tr	0.3	tr	tr	0	1	tr	1
0.5	0.1	tr	0.8	0.1	tr	0	3	tr	0
0.8	0.2	tr	**4.6**	0.6	**0.2**	0	20	6	0
0.5	0.1	0.1	2.7	0.4	0.1	tr	**32**	5	tr
0.7	0.1	tr	1.3	0.1	0.1	tr	4	1	tr
n	0.1	0.1	2.0	n	tr	tr	22	n	tr
0.5	0.1	0.1	1.8	0.3	0.1	0.7	7	4	1

SUGAR PRODUCTS

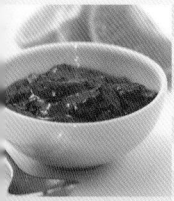

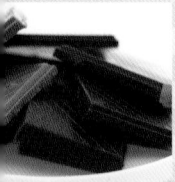

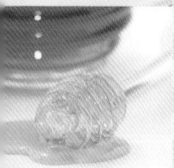

FOOD	AVERAGE PORTION SIZE	TOTAL CALORIES	FAT-SOLUBLE VITAMINS			
				A	D	
(where appropriate, numbers in brackets represent size of average portion)	grams per portion	kcals per portion	either Retinol (µg/portion) (QCT: 550µg/day)	or Carotene (µg/portion) (QCT: 3,300µg/day)	Cholecalciferol (µg/portion) (QCT: 0µg/day*)	*(*see pages 98–9)*
Sugars and syrups (1 tbs)						
Honey	20	**58**	0	0	0	
Molasses	20	**53**	0	0	0	
Sugar, brown	20	**72**	0	0	0	
Sugar, white	20	**79**	0	0	0	
Syrup, golden	20	**60**	0	0	0	
Syrup, maple	20	**52**	0	0	0	
Treacle, black	20	**51**	0	0	0	
Preserves and spreads (1 tbs)						
Chocolate nut spread	20	**110**	0	288	0	
Fruit spread	20	**24**	0	53	0	
Jam	20	**52**	0	46	0	
Marmalade	20	**52**	0	104	0	
Chocolate						
Chocolate bar (eg. Mars, Twix)	50	**221**	4	20	tr	
Milk chocolate	50	**260**	13	tr	0	
Plain chocolate	50	**255**	8	tr	0	
Confectionery						
Boiled sweets	50	**164**	0	0	0	
Cereal crunchy bar	50	**234**	0	tr	0	
Fruit pastilles	50	**164**	0	0	0	
Halva (with carrot)	50	**177**	**70**	**4,715**	**0.2**	
Liquorice shapes	50	**139**	0	0	0	
Nougat	50	**192**	0	10	0	
Peppermints	50	**197**	0	0	0	
Turkish delight (with nuts)	50	**172**	0	tr	0	

	WATER-SOLUBLE VITAMINS								
E	THE B-GROUP								C
Tocopherol (mg/portion) (QCT: 4mg/day)	Thiamin B1 (mg/portion) (QCT: 0.8mg/day)	Riboflavin B2 (mg/portion) (QCT: 1mg/day)	Niacin B3 (mg/portion) (QCT: 14mg/day)	Pantothenate B5 (mg/portion) (QCT: 5mg/day)	Pyridoxine B6 (mg/portion) (QCT: 1.3mg/day)	Cobalamin B12 (µg/portion) (QCT: 1µg/day)	Folate (µg/portion) (QCT: 150µg/day)	Biotin (µg/portion) (QCT: 30µg/day)	Ascorbic acid (mg/portion) (QCT: 30mg/day)
tr	tr	tr	tr	n	n	0	n	n	0
0.1	tr	tr	0.2	0	0.1	0	0	tr	0
0	tr	tr	tr	tr	tr	0	tr	tr	0
0	0	0	0	0	0	0	0	0	0
0	tr	tr	tr	0	tr	0	tr	tr	0
0	tr	tr	tr	tr	tr	0	0	tr	0
0	tr	tr	tr	tr	tr	0	tr	tr	0
0.5	0.1	tr	0.5	0.1	tr	0	3	n	tr
0.4	tr	tr	0.4	tr	tr	0	3	tr	1
0.6	tr	tr	0.3	0.1	tr	0	5	n	**2**
1.5	tr	tr	0.5	0.1	n	0	2	1	tr
0.5	tr	0.1	0.6	0.3	tr	tr	5	1	0
0.2	tr	**0.3**	1.4	**0.4**	tr	**0.5**	6	**2**	0
0.7	tr	tr	0.6	0.2	tr	0	6	**2**	0
0	0	0	0	0	0	0	0	0	0
1.9	0.1	0.1	**3.4**	n	0.1	0	**8**	n	tr
0	0	0	0	0	0	0	0	0	0
0.6	0.1	0.1	0.7	0.3	0.1	0	7	**2**	tr
0	0.1	tr	1.1	n	**0.3**	0	5	n	0
0.3	0.1	0.1	0.7	tr	tr	0	6	n	0
0	0	0	0	0	0	0	0	0	0
0.1	tr	tr	0.2	tr	0	0	2	tr	0

SOUPS AND SAUCES

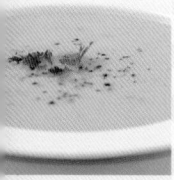

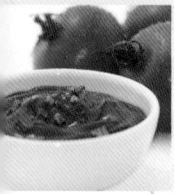

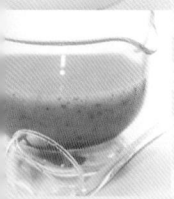

FOOD	AVERAGE PORTION SIZE	TOTAL CALORIES	FAT-SOLUBLE VITAMINS			
			A		D	
	grams/ml per portion	kcals per portion	either Retinol (µg/portion) (QCT: 550µg/day)	or Carotene (µg/portion) (QCT: 3,300µg/day)	Cholecalciferol (µg/portion) (QCT: 0µg/day*)	(*see pages 98–9)
Soups						
Bouillabaisse	250	**338**	tr	0	tr	
Carrot and orange soup	250	**50**	0	**2**	0	
Chicken soup	250	**145**	98	0	tr	
French onion soup	250	**100**	0	0	0	
Gazpacho	250	**113**	0	n	0	
Leek and potato soup	250	**130**	0	0	0	
Lentil soup	250	**293**	0	0	0	
Minestrone soup	250	**158**	33	0	tr	
Mushroom soup	250	**115**	100	0	0	
Oxtail soup	250	**110**	0	0	0	
Tomato soup	250	**130**	0	0	0	
Vegetable soup	250	**130**	0	1	0	
Sauces						
Black bean sauce	30	**28**	0	n	0	
Brown sauce (spicy)	30	**36**	0	tr	0	
Curry sauce	115	**90**	0	n	0	
Dressing, French	30	**139**	0	0	0	
Dressing, Thousand Island	30	**97**	4	0	0	
Dressing, yogurt-based	30	**88**	n	n	n	
Gravy (instant)	70	**24**	n	0	0	
Hollandaise sauce	70	**495**	**574**	0	**0.5**	
Mayonnaise	30	**207**	26	0	0	
Mint sauce	10	**10**	2	tr	0	
Raita	50	**29**	10	0	0	
Salad cream	30	**104**	tr	tr	0	
Soy sauce	10	**4**	0	0	0	
Sweet and sour sauce	150	**66**	0	n	0	
Tomato ketchup	30	**35**	0	0	0	

	WATER-SOLUBLE VITAMINS								
E	THE B-GROUP								C
Tocopherol (mg/portion) (QCT: 4mg/day)	Thiamin B1 (mg/portion) (QCT: 0.8mg/day)	Riboflavin B2 (mg/portion) (QCT: 1mg/day)	Niacin B3 (mg/portion) (QCT: 14mg/day)	Pantothenate B5 (mg/portion) (QCT: 5mg/day)	Pyridoxine B6 (mg/portion) (QCT: 1.3mg/day)	Cobalamin B12 (µg/portion) (QCT: 1µg/day)	Folate (µg/portion) (QCT: 150µg/day)	Biotin (µg/portion) (QCT: 30µg/day)	Ascorbic acid (mg/portion) (QCT: 30mg/day)
n	n	n	n	n	n	n	n	n	8
0.6	0.1	tr	0.5	0.3	0.1	0	10	tr	5
1.4	tr	0.1	1.3	0.1	tr	tr	3	0	0
0.4	0.1	tr	0.3	tr	0.1	0	5	3	13
2.3	0.1	tr	1.3	0.4	0.2	0	25	3	**28**
0.7	0.2	0.1	1.3	0.4	**0.3**	tr	**30**	3	8
n	0.2	0.1	1.3	**0.9**	**0.3**	0	15	n	3
0.8	0.1	tr	1.5	0.3	0.2	tr	23	tr	13
1.4	tr	0.1	1.3	0.3	tr	tr	5	3	0
0.5	0.1	0.1	**3.0**	0.1	0.1	0	3	0	0
3.5	0.1	0.1	1.5	0.3	0.2	tr	**30**	3	tr
0.6	0.2	tr	0.5	0.3	0.2	0	18	tr	8
n	**0.3**	tr	0.5	n	n	tr	n	n	tr
n	tr	tr	0.1	n	tr	0	2	n	tr
n	tr	tr	0.3	n	tr	0	n	n	0
n	0	0	0	tr	0	0	0	0	0
2.4	tr	tr	0.1	tr	tr	0	1	tr	tr
n	n	n	n	n	n	n	n	n	tr
n	n	n	n	n	n	0	0	n	0
1.7	tr	0.1	1.1	0.7	tr	**1.4**	12	**9**	0
5.7	tr	tr	0.1	n	tr	0.3	1	n	tr
tr	tr	tr	tr	tr	tr	0	tr	tr	tr
0	tr	0.1	0.6	0.2	tr	0	8	1	1
3.2	n	n	n	n	tr	0.3	1	n	0
n	tr	tr	0.5	n	n	0	1	n	0
n	0.2	tr	tr	n	n	0	n	n	n
n	**0.3**	tr	0.7	n	tr	0	tr	n	1

PICKLES AND SAVOURIES

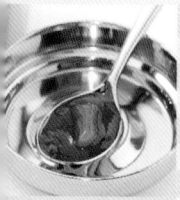

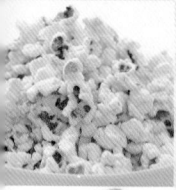

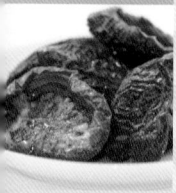

FOOD	AVERAGE PORTION SIZE	TOTAL CALORIES	FAT-SOLUBLE VITAMINS			
			A		D	
(where appropriate, numbers in brackets represent number of items in average portion)	grams per portion	kcals per portion	either Retinol (µg/portion) (QCT: 550µg/day)	or Carotene (µg/portion) (QCT: 3,300µg/day)	Cholecalciferol (µg/portion) (QCT: 0µg/day*)	*(*see pages 98–9)*
Pickles and chutneys						
Lime pickle	40	**71**	0	39	0	
Piccalilli	40	**34**	0	n	0	
Relish (corn/cucumber/onion)	40	**48**	0	n	0	
Sweet mango chutney	40	**76**	0	52	0	
Tomato chutney	40	**51**	0	156	0	
Tomatoes, sun-dried	50	**248**	0	**200**	0	
Savoury snacks						
Bombay mix	30	**164**	0	n	0	
Breadsticks (3)	20	**78**	0	tr	0	
Popcorn, plain	50	**297**	0	69	0	
Pork scratchings	25	**152**	0	0	tr	
Potato crisps	40	**212**	0	tr	0	
Potato crisps, low-fat	40	**183**	0	tr	0	
Pretzels	50	**191**	0	0	0	
Tortilla chips	50	**230**	0	114	0	
Twiglets	50	**192**	0	tr	0	

	WATER-SOLUBLE VITAMINS								
E	THE B-GROUP								C
Tocopherol (mg/portion) (QCT: 4mg/day)	Thiamin B1 (mg/portion) (QCT: 0.8mg/day)	Riboflavin B2 (mg/portion) (QCT: 1mg/day)	Niacin B3 (mg/portion) (QCT: 14mg/day)	Pantothenate B5 (mg/portion) (QCT: 5mg/day)	Pyridoxine B6 (mg/portion) (QCT: 1.3mg/day)	Cobalamin B12 (µg/portion) (QCT: 1µg/day)	Folate (µg/portion) (QCT: 150µg/day)	Biotin (µg/portion) (QCT: 30µg/day)	Ascorbic acid (mg/portion) (QCT: 30mg/day)
n	tr	tr	0.3	n	n	0	n	n	tr
n	tr	tr	0.1	n	tr	0	n	tr	tr
n	n	n	n	n	n	0	n	n	n
n	0	tr	0.4	n	n	0	n	n	tr
0.4	tr	0.1	0.4	0.1	0.1	0	7	1	2
12.0	n	n	n	n	n	0	n	n	tr
n	0.1	0.1	**4.3**	0.3	0.1	0	26	tr	tr
0.1	tr	tr	1.1	0.1	tr	tr	4	tr	0
3.3	0.1	tr	0.5	0.1	0.1	0	3	1	0
n	**0.2**	0.1	2.0	n	tr	n	n	n	0
2.3	0.1	tr	1.8	0.4	**0.3**	0	15	n	2
1.4	0.1	0.1	2.6	n	0.2	0	19	n	**6**
n	**0.2**	**0.3**	2.7	0.1	0.1	0	n	n	0
1.0	0.1	tr	0.9	n	0.2	0	10	n	tr
1.2	**0.2**	0.2	3.9	**0.8**	0.2	0	**39**	**8**	tr

DRINKS

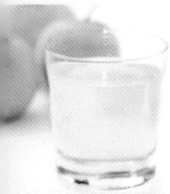

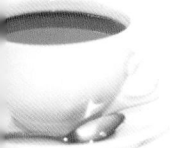

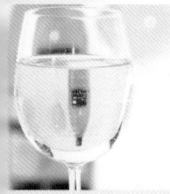

FOOD	AVERAGE PORTION SIZE	TOTAL CALORIES	FAT-SOLUBLE VITAMINS			
			A		D	
(where appropriate, numbers in brackets represent size of average portion)	ml per portion	kcals per portion	either Retinol (µg/portion) (QCT: 550µg/day)	or Carotene (µg/portion) (QCT: 3,300µg/day)	Cholecalciferol (µg/portion) (QCT: 0µg/day*)	*(*see pages 98–9)*
Fruit juices (unsweetened)						
Apple juice	200	**76**	0	tr	0	
Cranberry juice	200	**122**	0	42	**5.6**	
Grape juice	200	**92**	0	tr	0	
Grapefruit juice	200	**66**	0	tr	0	
Lemon juice	20	**1**	0	tr	0	
Lime juice	20	**2**	0	tr	0	
Mango juice (canned)	200	**78**	0	420	0	
Orange juice	200	**66**	0	34	0	
Passion fruit juice	200	**94**	0	1,600	0	
Pineapple juice	200	**82**	0	16	0	
Pomegranate juice	200	**88**	0	66	0	
Prune juice	200	**114**	0	n	0	
Hot drinks						
Coffee, black	190	**4**	0	0	0	
Coffee, with milk	190	**13**	11	2	tr	
Coffee, Irish	190	**160**	n	101	tr	
Drinking chocolate (for 1 mug)	18	**66**	0	n	0	
Horlicks (for 1 mug)	24	**95**	**112**	n	0.4	
Ovaltine (for 1 mug)	24	**91**	n	n	n	
Tea, black	190	**tr**	0	0	0	
Tea, with milk	190	**15**	11	tr	0	
Tea, green	190	**tr**	0	0	0	
Tea, herbal	190	**2**	n	0	0	
Soft drinks (carbonated)						
Cola	330	**129**	0	0	0	
Fruit juice drink (eg. Tango)	330	**129**	0	310	0	
Ginger ale	250	**38**	0	0	0	
Lemonade	200	**44**	0	tr	0	

continues

	WATER-SOLUBLE VITAMINS								
E	THE B-GROUP								C
Tocopherol (mg/portion) (QCT: 4mg/day)	Thiamin B1 (mg/portion) (QCT: 0.8mg/day)	Riboflavin B2 (mg/portion) (QCT: 1mg/day)	Niacin B3 (mg/portion) (QCT: 14mg/day)	Pantothenate B5 (mg/portion) (QCT: 5mg/day)	Pyridoxine B6 (mg/portion) (QCT: 1.3mg/day)	Cobalamin B12 (µg/portion) (QCT: 1µg/day)	Folate (µg/portion) (QCT: 150µg/day)	Biotin (µg/portion) (QCT: 30µg/day)	Ascorbic acid (mg/portion) (QCT: 30mg/day)
tr	tr	tr	0.2	0.1	tr	0	8	2	28
1.1	**2.4**	**3.4**	**42.2**	1.0	**4.4**	**4**	**600**	6	0
tr	tr	tr	0.2	0.1	0.1	0	2	1	tr
0.4	0.1	tr	0.4	0.2	tr	0	12	2	62
n	tr	tr	tr	tr	tr	0	3	tr	7
n	tr	tr	tr	tr	tr	0	n	n	8
2.1	tr	tr	1.0	n	n	0	n	n	50
0.3	0.2	tr	0.6	0.3	0.1	0	56	2	96
n	tr	0.1	1.6	n	n	0	n	n	42
0.1	0.1	tr	0.4	0.1	0.1	0	16	tr	22
n	tr	0.1	0.4	**1.1**	0.6	0	n	n	16
n	tr	0.1	1.4	n	0.3	0	tr	n	tr
tr	tr	tr	1.3	tr	tr	0	tr	**6**	0
tr	0.1	tr	1.3	0.1	tr	tr	2	**6**	0
0.3	0.1	0.1	1.0	0.1	tr	tr	2	4	0
tr	tr	tr	0.4	n	tr	0	2	n	0
tr	0.2	0.3	3.4	n	n	n	n	n	0
tr	0.4	n	0.5	n	n	n	n	n	0
n	tr	tr	0	0.1	tr	0	6	2	0
tr	0	0.1	0	0.1	tr	tr	6	2	0
n	0	tr	0.2	tr	tr	0	tr	tr	6
n	tr	tr	0	tr	0	0	2	0	0
0	0	0	0	0	0	0	0	0	0
tr	tr	tr	tr	tr	tr	0	3	tr	3
0	0	0	0	0	0	0	0	0	0
tr	0	0	0	tr	tr	0	tr	tr	tr

DRINKS

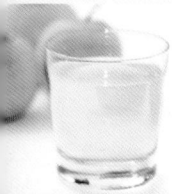

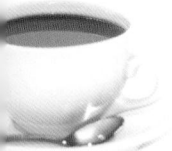

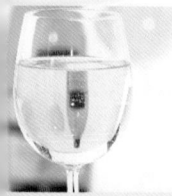

FOOD	AVERAGE PORTION SIZE	TOTAL CALORIES	FAT-SOLUBLE VITAMINS			
			A		D	
	ml per portion	kcals per portion	either Retinol (µg/portion) (QCT: 550µg/day)	or Carotene (µg/portion) (QCT: 3,300µg/day)	Cholecalciferol (µg/portion) (QCT: 0µg/day*)	*(*see pages 98–9)*
Lucozade	200	**120**	0	**1,670**	0	
Tonic water	250	**83**	0	0	0	
Soft drinks (uncarbonated)						
Barley water (diluted)	200	**28**	0	250	0	
Ribena (diluted)	200	**60**	0	n	0	
Fruit juice drink (diluted)	200	**74**	0	n	0	
Rosehip syrup (diluted)	200	**92**	0	200	0	
Alcoholic drinks						
Beer, bitter	300	**177**	0	tr	0	
Beer, lager	300	**384**	0	tr	0	
Beer, shandy	300	**48**	0	tr	0	
Beer, stout	300	**156**	0	tr	0	
Cider	300	**108**	0	tr	0	
Champagne	125	**95**	0	tr	0	
Red wine	125	**85**	0	tr	0	
White wine	125	**83**	0	tr	0	
Port	50	**79**	0	tr	0	
Sherry	50	**58**	0	tr	0	
Vermouth/martini	50	**55**	0	tr	0	
Cream liqueurs (eg. Baileys)	25	**81**	48	23	tr	
Liqueurs, high-strength (eg. pernod)	25	**79**	0	tr	0	
Liqueurs, med.-strength (eg. campari)	25	**66**	0	tr	0	
Spirits (eg. brandy/gin/whisky)	25	**56**	0	0	0	

	WATER-SOLUBLE VITAMINS								
E	THE B-GROUP								C
Tocopherol (mg/portion) (QCT: 4mg/day)	Thiamin B1 (mg/portion) (QCT: 0.8mg/day)	Riboflavin B2 (mg/portion) (QCT: 1mg/day)	Niacin B3 (mg/portion) (QCT: 14mg/day)	Pantothenate B5 (mg/portion) (QCT: 5mg/day)	Pyridoxine B6 (mg/portion) (QCT: 1.3mg/day)	Cobalamin B12 (µg/portion) (QCT: 1µg/day)	Folate (µg/portion) (QCT: 150µg/day)	Biotin (µg/portion) (QCT: 30µg/day)	Ascorbic acid (mg/portion) (QCT: 30mg/day)
0	0	0	0	tr	tr	0	2	tr	16
0	0	0	0	0	0	0	0	0	0
n	0	0	tr	0	0	0	0	0	4
n	0	0	2.0	0	0.3	0	0	0	20
n	tr	tr	0.2	tr	tr	0	4	tr	14
0	0	0	0	0	0	0	0	0	**118**
n	tr	0.1	1.2	0.3	0.2	tr	9	3	0
n	tr	0.1	3.0	0.1	0.2	tr	36	3	0
n	tr	tr	0.3	0.1	tr	tr	3	tr	0
n	tr	0.1	3.0	0.1	tr	tr	18	3	0
n	tr	tr	0	0.1	tr	tr	n	3	0
n	tr	tr	0.1	tr	tr	tr	tr	n	0
n	tr	tr	0.1	0.1	tr	tr	1	3	0
n	tr	tr	0	tr	tr	tr	tr	n	0
0	tr	tr	tr	n	tr	tr	tr	n	0
0	tr	tr	tr	n	tr	tr	tr	n	0
0	tr	tr	0	n	tr	tr	tr	n	0
0.1	n	n	n	n	n	0	tr	n	0
0	tr	tr	tr	tr	tr	tr	tr	tr	0
0	tr	tr	tr	tr	tr	tr	tr	tr	0
0	0	0	0	0	0	0	0	0	0

All about minerals

CALCIUM

Calcium gives strength to bones and teeth, which together contain 99 per cent of the calcium in the body. It is also important for the health of the heart, muscles and nerves, and is a component of various enzymes and hormones. Calcium is abundant in food, and is also found in hard drinking water.

The skeleton acts like a calcium "bank", ensuring that there is always enough available to support vital functions. "Deposits" and "withdrawals" are controlled by hormones,

Calcium TOP 10 (milligrams per 100 grams of food)

World Health Organisation recommended intake = 500 mg/day
Toxicity level = not defined

1.	parmesan cheese	1025	7.	purple-sprouting broccoli	200
2.	sesame seeds	670	8.	okra, chick peas, brazil nuts	160
3.	tofu	510	9.	spring greens, spinach, curly kale	170
4.	cheese (on average)	450	10.	milk	130
5.	anchovies, sardines	420			
6.	dried figs, almonds, yogurt	250			

including parathyroid and thyroid hormones, calcitonin, growth hormone, sex hormones, cortisone and insulin. If dietary calcium is lacking, or there is a problem with absorption, the calcium bank account may become overdrawn causing problems such as tooth decay, osteoporosis, osteomalacia and rickets.

Calcium absorption from food depends on the presence of vitamin D, and is influenced by lifestyle choices including diet, alcohol intake, smoking and exercise. The amount absorbed depends on availability and how much is circulating in the blood.

Too much calcium in the bloodstream – usually the result of excessive calcium supplements or indigestion remedies – causes nausea, depression and even kidney stones and kidney damage. High calcium intakes are sometimes recommended for osteoporosis, but there is no firm evidence that this is effective.

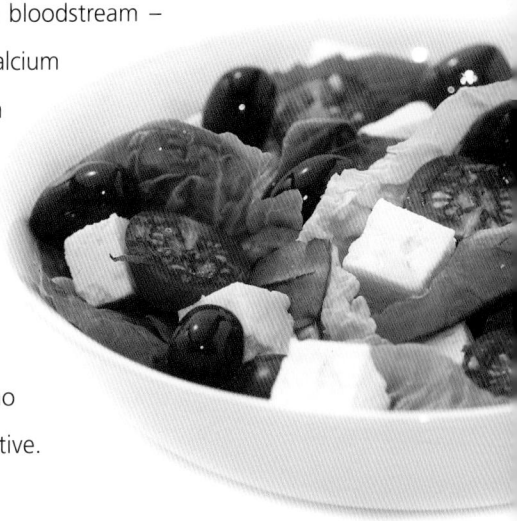

Magnesium TOP 10 (milligrams per 100 grams of food)

World Health Organisation recommended intake = 200 mg/day
Toxicity level = not defined

1.	brazil nuts	410	6.	beans (on average)	110
2.	sesame seeds, sunflower seeds	380	7.	swiss chard, spinach, okra	75
3.	winkles	310	8.	anchovies, sardines, crab, prawns	50
4.	almonds, cashews, pine nuts	270	9.	cheddar cheese	39
5.	walnuts	160	10.	meat, fish (on average)	25

MAGNESIUM

Magnesium is found in most foods and after calcium is the second most abundant mineral in the body. It helps to maintain healthy bones and teeth, and protects against epilepsy, hypertension, heart disease, osteoporosis, premenstrual tension and mental disturbance. Magnesium assists vitamin B1 in releasing energy from carbohydrates, alcohol and fats, and vitamin B6 in the metabolism of protein. It is also needed for calcium absorption. Excess calcium in the diet reduces magnesium absorption.

It is difficult to say how much dietary magnesium is necessary because the body only absorbs what it needs at any given time, regardless of availability. If dietary magnesium is low, absorption becomes more efficient (and less is excreted by the kidneys) in order to maintain magnesium levels in the blood.

Diarrhoea, diabetes, alcoholism and diuretic drugs can all cause magnesium deficiency. Symptoms of deficiency include muscle cramps and spasms. Low intake may also be related to high blood pressure. Excess dietary magnesium may cause diarrhoea, but magnesium toxicity is rare and usually only occurs in cases of kidney failure. The first signs of toxicity are thirst and flushing, followed by falling blood pressure.

Phosphorus TOP 10 (milligrams per 100 grams of food)

World Health Organisation recommended intake = 550 mg/day
Toxicity level = not defined

1.	wheat bran	1200	7.	dried beans, lentils, chick peas	350
2.	yeast extract	950	8.	muesli	280
3.	nuts, seeds, soya beans (on average)	680	9.	fish, shellfish (on average)	250
4.	sardines	540	10.	eggs, meat (on average)	200
5.	cheese (on average)	500			
6.	pearl barley, rye flour, self-raising flour	400			

PHOSPHORUS

Phosphorus forms part of the structure of proteins, carbohydrates and fats and is therefore present in all foods. In the body it is an important component of bones and teeth, and is also found in the chemical adenosine tri-phosphate (ATP), which is vital for the release of the energy contained in the food we eat.

A proper balance between phosphorus and calcium in the body is necessary for health. The kidneys play a central role in maintaining this balance by controlling the amount of phosphorus lost in the urine. However, it is also important to balance these two minerals in the diet. This is particularly the case with children and infants, who have smaller and more sensitive bodies than adults – too much phosphorus in a baby's diet (for example, from unprocessed cows' milk) can cause muscle spasms.

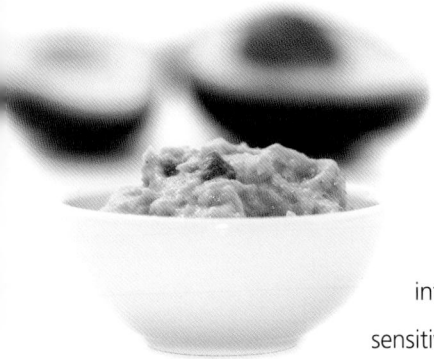

Phosphorus deficiency is very rare, but pregnancy, vitamin D deficiency, serious injury, some drugs and alcoholism can all cause phosphorus levels to fall. This lowers immunity and may

Potassium TOP 10 (milligrams per 100 grams of food)

World Health Organisation recommended intake = 2000 mg/day
Toxicity level = 18 g/day

1.	yeast extract	2100	7.	sweet potato, avocado, greens, cabbages	450
2.	dried apricots	1880	8.	banana	400
3.	wheat bran, wheat germ	1050	9.	potato, endive, courgette	360
4.	beans, peas, lentils	1000	10.	meat and fish (on average)	350
5.	dried fruit	900			
6.	nuts (on average)	750			

lead to muscle weakness and softening of the bones (osteomalacia). In children, deficiency may produce retarded growth.

POTASSIUM

Potassium boosts energy and strength, and enables nerves and muscles to function properly. It is also involved in the regulation of blood-sugar levels. Eating a diet rich in potassium helps the body to get rid of excess sodium, which in turn helps to prevent high blood pressure. Fresh fruits and vegetables contain more potassium than sodium, whereas processed fast foods and meat contain more sodium than potassium. Too much sodium in the diet (in the form of added salt) may reduce potassium levels in the body.

Potassium deficiency can be caused by gastrointestinal disorders, diabetes, diuretics, steroids and laxatives. It produces a variety of symptoms, including poor appetite, tiredness, depression, constipation, palpitations, muscle weakness, cramps and, in severe cases, heart failure. Potassium overload can result from excessive potassium supplements and is also caused by severe dehydration and kidney or adrenal failure. High blood levels of potassium are very toxic and lead to rapid heart failure.

SODIUM AND CHLORIDE

In nature, sodium and chloride are usually found bound together into salt, a condiment long treasured for its flavour-enhancing properties. Together with potassium, both minerals play a major role in maintaining the water balance in the body, and sodium is also important for nerve and muscle function.

Excessive sweating, burns, severe vomiting, diarrhoea, diuretic therapy and kidney damage can all cause loss of salt and water from the body. This leads to dehydration accompanied by nausea, dizziness, vomiting, muscle cramps and exhaustion. Unless treated by the replacement of water and salt, dehydration may lead to life-threatening shock.

In affluent societies, however, excess salt causes health problems. The amount of salt needed is only a fraction of the amount routinely eaten and high blood pressure and heart disease are clearly associated with excessive salt intake.

The easiest way to reduce salt intake is to eat a diet based on fresh fruits and vegetables, and to cut down on fast foods, processed meats and snacks. Since much of the salt we eat is incorporated into food, it is more effective to change what we eat rather than to reduce our consumption of table salt.

Sodium Chloride TOP 10 (milligrams per 100 grams of food)

World Health Organisation recommended intake = <3900 mg/day
Toxicity level = depends on individual circumstances

1.	anchovies	3930
2.	seaweed	2500
3.	olives	2250
4.	bacon	1960
5.	smoked salmon	1880
6.	salami	1800
7.	tomato ketchup, sweet pickle, brown sauce	1630
8.	prawns	1590
9.	feta cheese, Danish blue cheese	1330
10.	Twiglets, pot savouries	1320

All about trace elements

IRON

The body contains iron in red blood cells, muscles, enzymes and liver stores. It is used for transporting oxygen around the body, for hormone and bile production, for releasing energy from food and in the elimination of toxins and waste products.

Iron exists in food in two forms – haem and non-haem. Animal-based foods contain haem iron, which is easier to absorb. Plant foods contain non-haem iron, in addition to other nutrients, such as vitamin C, which increase iron absorption. Whatever the iron content of the diet, absorption rates change according to whether body stores are depleted or full.

Worldwide, iron deficiency is a common consequence of malnutrition. In developed countries, blood loss or inhibited absorption (caused by excessive intake of tea, fibre, milk, soya or calcium supplements) are more likely causes. Deficiency leads to anaemia, causing breathlessness, palpitations, dizziness, persistent tiredness, mood changes and poor concentration.

Iron overload, usually the result of taking supplements, causes stomach pain and constipation. Frequent iron injections,

Iron Top 10 (milligrams per 100 grams of food)

World Health Organisation recommended intake = 9 mg/day (for men); 12.5 mg/day (for women)
Toxicity level = 20 mg/kg of body weight in one dose

1.	cockles	28.0	6.	fresh mint	9.5
2.	Bran Flakes and Special K	24.3	7.	kidney	9.0
3.	wheat bran, Weetabix	12.9	8.	beans, chick peas, lentils, wheat germ	8.3
4.	liver	11.3	9.	fresh parsley	7.7
5.	sesame seeds, pumpkin seeds	10.4	10.	dried peaches	6.8

blood transfusions, various blood and liver disorders, and haemochromatosis (a hereditary disease) can also produce toxic overload, leading to heart failure and liver damage.

ZINC

Zinc is essential for growth, blood fat regulation and protein, carbohydrate and alcohol metabolism. It promotes wound healing, the elimination of waste from working muscles and insulin and seminal fluid production. It also protects against prostate disease and mental disturbance.

Zinc absorption is improved by vitamin B6, while excess calcium and some food additives inhibit it. Health problems such as sudden weight loss, alcohol abuse, gastrointestinal disorders, burns and surgery cause zinc deficiency, and a typical fast food diet – high in fat and refined carbohydrate – is low in zinc.

Symptoms of deficiency include loss of appetite, diarrhoea, skin problems, poor wound healing, lowered immunity, loss of taste and smell, hair loss, white spots on the nails, tiredness, mental disturbance and "pica" (eating dirt) in children. Too much zinc, usually from supplements, causes nausea and vomiting, and may interfere with copper, iron and calcium absorption.

Zinc TOP 10 (milligrams per 100 grams of food)

World Health Organisation recommended intake = 9.4 mg/day
Toxicity level = 2 g in a single dose; 50 mg/day, long-term

1.	wheat germ, bran	17.0	7.	cod roe	3.3
2.	liver	15.9	8.	wholemeal pasta, beans, chick peas	3.0
3.	whelks	12.1	9.	anchovies, sardines, shellfish	2.5
4.	nuts, seeds	5.3	10.	oatcakes	2.3
5.	soya beans, lentils	4.0			
6.	kidney, meat, cheese	3.5			

MANGANESE

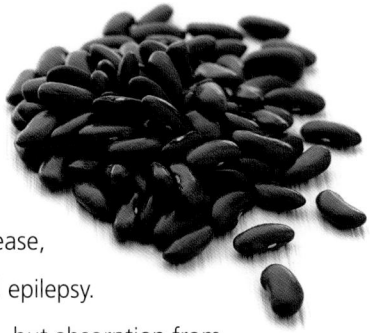

Manganese is vital for healthy bones. It is also involved in protein, fat and cholesterol metabolism, preserving cell membranes and preventing heart disease, cancer, rheumatoid arthritis, diabetes and epilepsy.

Severe deficiency is virtually unknown, but absorption from the gut is inhibited by the presence of calcium, phosphorus and zinc. Mild deficiency has been linked with cancer, myasthenia gravis, rheumatoid arthritis, diabetes, atherosclerosis, heart disease, epilepsy and schizophrenia. Excess manganese – from

Manganese TOP 10 (milligrams per 100 grams of food)

Safe intake = 1–10 mg/day

1.	dried sage	25.0	8.	muesli, chick peas, soya beans	2.6
2.	wheat germ	12.3	9.	peanuts, coconut, cashews, almonds, sunflower seeds, sesame seeds	2.0
3.	wheat bran	9.0	10.	blackberries, lentils, tempeh, tofu	1.3
4.	pine nuts	7.9			
5.	macadamia nuts, hazelnuts, pecans	5.2			
6.	oyster mushrooms	3.6			
7.	walnuts	3.4			

taking supplements or in drinking water – may cause psychosis and a neurological condition resembling Parkinson's disease.

COPPER

Copper helps to keep red blood cells healthy and may protect against osteoporosis and arthritis. Deficiency is uncommon but occurs in cases of malnutrition, malabsorption and chronic diarrhoea. Zinc, cadmium, fluoride and molybdenum supplements may inhibit absorption. Symptoms of deficiency include anaemia, osteoporosis, lowered immunity, de-pigmentation, poor growth and hypothyroidism.

Copper TOP 10 (milligrams per 100 grams of food)

World Health Organisation recommended intake = 1.15 mg/day
Toxicity level = uncertain

1.	calf liver	23.86	6.	cashew nuts	2.11
2.	lamb liver	13.54	7.	brazil nuts	1.76
3.	whelks	6.59	8.	winkles	1.70
4.	ox liver, pig liver	2.40	9.	soya beans, crab, lobster	1.50
5.	sunflower seeds, melon seeds	2.30	10.	sesame seeds, pumpkin seeds	1.48

Iodine TOP 10 (micrograms per 100 grams of food)

World Health Organisation recommended intake = 150 μg/day
Toxicity level = 1000 μg/day

1.	dried seaweed, kombu	448670	6.	–, nori	1470
2.	–, arame	84140	7.	cockles, mussels	140
3.	–, hijiki	42670	8.	cod, lobster	100
4.	–, wakame	16830	9.	kipper, yogurt, eggs	63
5.	–, dulse	5970	10.	salmon, butter, milk, cheese	31

iodized salt contains 3100 μg
sea salt contains 50 μg

IODINE

Iodine is a vital component of the thyroid hormones that regulate metabolism and tissue repair, and promote growth and development. Iodine deficiency is uncommon in developed countries but is a problem in developing parts of the world causing goitre (enlarged thyroid) and thyroid underactivity. This results in weight gain, lethargy, constipation, dry skin and hair, and (sometimes) mental disturbance. Iodine deficiency may also cause retarded growth and impaired mental development in children. A high intake of iodine causes thyroid dysfunction.

SELENIUM

Selenium is an antioxidant, which boosts immunity and helps red blood cells to function properly. The amount of selenium in plants depends on how much they absorb from the soil so the amount of selenium in food is very variable. Pollution and intensive farming have reduced soil selenium levels and food processing methods also reduce the selenium content in food.

Deficiency lowers immunity and is linked with cancer, heart disease, stroke, eye disease and male infertility. Severe deficiency in young people causes degenerative heart disease. Supplement overdose may cause hair loss, brittle nails, itchy skin rash and, in severe cases, neurological disturbance and paralysis.

Selenium TOP 10 (micrograms per 100 grams of food)

World Health Organisation recommended intake = 40 µg/day
Toxicity level = 6 µg/kg/day

1.	brazil nuts	254	6.	liver	50
2.	kidney	209	7.	sunflower seeds	49
3.	lentils	105	8.	mussels	43
4.	tuna	78	9.	sardines, plaice, kipper, mackerel	39
5.	squid, lemon sole, lobster	62	10.	cashew nuts	34

MINERAL AND TRACE ELEMENT TABLES

These tables give the calorie, mineral and trace element contents of a wide selection of foods. The minerals listed are calcium, magnesium, phosphorus, potassium and sodium chloride. The trace elements are iron, zinc, manganese, copper, iodine and selenium. The calorie, mineral and trace element contents of each food are given "per average portion" rather than "per 100 grams". This allows you to work out the nutrient content of your diet without using weights or measures.

To find out how rich a food is in a particular mineral or trace element, compare the amount contained in a single portion ("n" is given where the figure is not known; "tr" denotes trace) with the Quality Calorie Target (QCT) given at the top of the column. This will enable you to assess your daily intake, and help you choose foods that will boost your intake of particular minerals and trace elements. The figures in bold denote the foods with the highest nutrient scores in each food category.

FRUIT

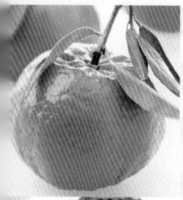

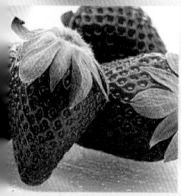

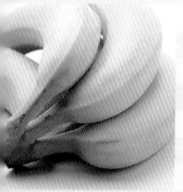

FOOD	AVERAGE PORTION SIZE	TOTAL CALORIES	MINERALS	
(where appropriate, numbers in brackets represent number of fruit in average portion)	grams per portion	kcals per portion	Calcium (mg/portion) (QCT: 500mg/day)	Magnesium (mg/portion) (QCT: 200mg/day)
Fresh fruit				
Apple (1)	100	**47**	4	5
Apricot (2)	130	**40**	20	14
Date (4)	100	**124**	24	24
Fig (2)	110	**47**	42	17
Grapes (bunch)	100	**60**	13	7
Kiwi fruit (2)	120	**59**	30	18
Melon (all types) (1 slice)	180	**43**	25	20
Peach/nectarine (1)	150	**55**	11	15
Pear (1)	170	**68**	19	12
Plum/greengage (2)	100	**39**	17	8
Rhubarb	100	**7**	93	13
Sharon fruit (1)	110	**80**	11	12
Tropical fruit				
Banana (1)	100	**95**	6	34
Guava (1)	140	**36**	18	17
Lychee (5)	75	**44**	5	7
Mango (½)	180	**103**	22	23
Papaya/paw-paw (¼)	140	**50**	32	15
Passion fruit (5)	75	**27**	8	22
Pineapple (2 slices)	160	**66**	29	26
Pomegranate (1)	100	**51**	12	11
Citrus fruit				
Clementine/satsuma/tangerine (2)	120	**43**	37	12
Grapefruit/pomelo, pink (1)	180	**54**	41	16
Lemon/lime (1)	100	**12**	25	10
Orange (1)	160	**59**	75	16
Berries				
Blackberries (20)	100	**25**	41	23
Blackcurrants	100	**28**	60	17

continues

MINERALS			TRACE ELEMENTS					
Phosphorus (mg/portion) (QCT: 550mg/day)	Potassium (mg/portion) (QCT: 2000mg/day)	Sodium Chloride (mg/portion) (max: 3900mg/day)	Copper (mg/portion) (QCT: 1.15mg/day)	Iron (mg/portion) (QCT: 9–12.5mg/day)	Iodine (µg/portion) (QCT: 150µg/day)	Manganese (mg/portion) (QCT: 1.4mg/day)	Selenium (µg/portion) (QCT: 40µg/day)	Zinc (mg/portion) (QCT: 9.4mg/day)
11	120	3	0.02	0.1	tr	0.1	tr	0.1
26	351	3	0.08	0.7	tr	0.1	1	0.1
28	410	7	0.12	0.3	n	0.2	1	0.2
17	220	3	0.07	0.3	n	0.1	tr	0.3
18	210	2	0.12	0.3	1	0.1	1	0.1
38	348	5	0.16	0.5	n	0.1	n	0.1
23	342	43	tr	0.4	n	tr	tr	tr
33	255	2	0.09	0.6	5	0.2	tr	0.2
22	255	5	0.10	0.3	2	tr	tr	0.2
23	310	2	0.10	0.4	tr	0.1	tr	0.1
17	290	3	0.07	0.3	n	0.2	tr	0.1
21	231	6	0.11	0.1	n	0.3	n	0.1
28	400	1	0.10	0.3	8	0.4	1	0.2
35	322	7	0.14	0.6	n	0.1	n	0.3
23	120	1	0.11	0.4	n	0.1	n	0.2
29	324	4	0.22	1.3	n	0.5	n	0.2
18	280	7	0.11	0.7	n	0.1	n	0.3
48	158	14	n	1.0	n	n	n	0.6
16	256	3	0.18	0.3	tr	0.8	tr	0.2
29	240	2	0.17	0.7	n	n	n	0.4
22	156	5	0.01	0.1	n	tr	n	0.1
36	360	5	0.04	0.2	n	tr	2	tr
18	130	2	0.05	0.4	n	tr	n	0.1
34	240	8	0.08	0.2	3	tr	2	0.2
31	160	2	0.11	0.7	n	1.4	tr	0.2
43	120	3	0.14	1.3	n	0.3	n	0.3

FRUIT

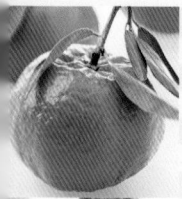

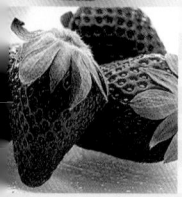

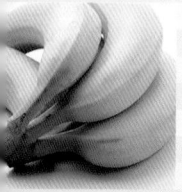

FOOD	AVERAGE PORTION SIZE	TOTAL CALORIES	MINERALS	
(where appropriate, numbers in brackets represent number of fruit in average portion)	grams per portion	kcals per portion	Calcium (mg/portion) (QCT: 500mg/day)	Magnesium (mg/portion) (QCT: 200mg/day)
Blueberries (bilberries)	100	**30**	12	5
Cherries (10)	100	**48**	13	10
Cranberries	100	**15**	12	7
Elderberries	100	**35**	37	n
Gooseberries	100	**40**	19	9
Raspberries (25)	100	**25**	25	19
Redcurrants	100	**21**	36	13
Strawberries (10)	120	**32**	19	12
Dried fruit				
Apricot (10)	100	**132**	92	65
Date (6)	100	**203**	45	41
Fig (5)	100	**227**	**250**	80
Pear (10 slices)	100	**207**	55	35
Pineapple (6 slices)	100	**276**	120	**110**
Prune (10)	100	**160**	38	27
Raisins and sultanas (3 tbs)	100	**163**	46	35

MINERALS			TRACE ELEMENTS					
Phosphoros (mg/portion) (QCT: 550mg/day)	Potassium (mg/portion) (QCT: 2000mg/day)	Sodium Chloride (mg/portion) (max: 3900mg/day)	Copper (mg/portion) (QCT: 1.15mg/day)	Iron (mg/portion) (QCT: 9–12.5mg/day)	Iodine (µg/portion) (QCT: 150µg/day)	Manganese (mg/portion) (QCT: 1.4mg/day)	Selenium (µg/portion) (QCT: 40µg/day)	Zinc (mg/portion) (QCT: 9.4mg/day)
14	88	3	0.08	0.5	n	0.3	tr	0.2
21	210	1	0.07	0.2	tr	0.1	1	0.1
11	95	2	0.05	0.7	n	0.1	n	0.2
48	290	1	n	1.6	n	n	n	n
19	170	1	0.06	0.6	tr	0.1	tr	0.1
31	170	3	0.10	0.7	n	0.4	n	0.3
30	280	2	0.12	1.2	n	0.2	n	0.2
29	192	7	0.08	0.5	**11**	0.4	tr	0.1
120	**1,880**	56	0.40	4.1	n	0.4	7	**0.7**
60	700	10	0.26	1.3	n	0.3	3	0.4
89	970	**62**	0.30	**4.2**	n	0.5	tr	0.7
65	750	15	0.30	1.0	5	0.2	2	0.5
65	1,080	15	**0.74**	1.3	tr	**3.4**	tr	**0.7**
83	860	12	0.16	2.9	n	0.3	3	0.5
76	1,020	60	0.39	3.8	n	0.3	**8**	**0.7**

NUTS AND SEEDS

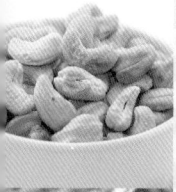

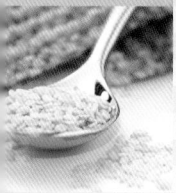

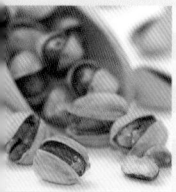

FOOD	AVERAGE PORTION SIZE	TOTAL CALORIES	MINERALS	
	grams per portion	kcals per portion	Calcium (mg/portion) (QCT: 500mg/day)	Magnesium (mg/portion) (QCT: 200mg/day)
Almonds	50	**306**	120	135
Brazil nuts	50	**341**	85	205
Cashew nuts	50	**287**	16	135
Chestnuts, dried	50	**160**	10	6
Coconut, fresh	100	**351**	13	41
Coconut, desiccated	50	**302**	12	45
Hazelnuts	50	**325**	70	80
Macadamia nuts (salted)	50	**374**	24	50
Melon seeds	50	**292**	36	**255**
Peanuts	50	**282**	30	105
Peanut butter	20	**125**	7	36
Pecan nuts	50	**345**	31	65
Pine nuts	50	**344**	6	135
Pistachio nuts (salted)	50	**301**	55	65
Pumpkin seeds	50	**285**	20	135
Sesame seeds	50	**299**	335	185
Sesame spread (tahini)	50	**304**	**340**	190
Sunflower seeds	50	**291**	55	195
Walnuts	50	**344**	47	80

MINERALS			TRACE ELEMENTS					
Phosphorus (mg/portion) (QCT: 550mg/day)	Potassium (mg/portion) (QCT: 2000mg/day)	Sodium Chloride (mg/portion) (max: 3900mg/day)	Copper (mg/portion) (QCT: 1.15mg/day)	Iron (mg/portion) (QCT: 9–12.5mg/day)	Iodine (µg/portion) (QCT: 150µg/day)	Manganese (mg/portion) (QCT: 1.4mg/day)	Selenium (µg/portion) (QCT: 40µg/day)	Zinc (mg/portion) (QCT: 9.4mg/day)
275	390	7	0.50	1.5	1	0.9	2	1.6
295	330	2	0.88	1.3	**10**	0.6	**765**	2.1
280	355	8	1.06	3.1	6	0.9	15	3.0
26	190	33	0.01	0.5	3	0.4	1	0.2
94	370	17	0.32	2.1	1	1.0	3	0.5
80	330	14	0.28	1.8	2	0.9	2	0.5
150	365	3	0.62	1.6	9	2.5	tr	1.1
100	150	140	0.22	0.8	n	2.8	4	0.6
345	325	50	**1.20**	3.8	n	1.2	n	2.0
215	335	1	0.51	1.3	**10**	1.1	2	1.8
66	140	70	0.14	0.4	n	0.3	1	0.6
155	260	1	0.54	1.1	n	2.3	6	2.7
325	390	1	0.66	2.8	n	**4.0**	n	**3.3**
210	**520**	**265**	0.42	1.5	n	0.5	3	3.0
425	410	9	0.79	5.0	n	n	n	**3.3**
360	285	10	0.73	5.2	n	0.8	n	2.7
365	290	10	0.74	**5.3**	n	0.8	n	2.7
320	355	2	1.14	3.2	n	1.1	25	2.6
190	225	4	0.67	1.5	5	1.7	10	1.4

VEGETABLES AND PULSES

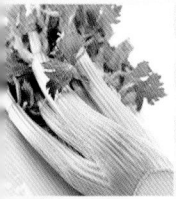

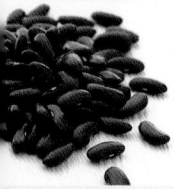

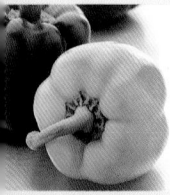

FOOD	AVERAGE PORTION SIZE	TOTAL CALORIES	MINERALS	
	grams per portion	kcals per portion	Calcium (mg/portion) (QCT: 500mg/day)	Magnesium (mg/portion) (QCT: 200mg/day)
Root vegetables				
Beetroot	100	**36**	20	11
Carrot	100	**35**	25	3
Celeriac	100	**18**	40	21
Parsnip	100	**64**	41	23
Potato, baked	180	**245**	20	58
Potato, boiled in salted water	180	**130**	9	25
Potato, mashed	180	**187**	22	23
Potato, chips (all types, average)	180	**398**	20	45
Swede	100	**24**	53	9
Sweet potato, baked	130	**150**	40	30
Beans, peas and lentils				
Aduki beans, cooked	100	**123**	39	60
Baked beans, in tomato sauce	130	**105**	62	40
Bean sprouts, fresh	60	**19**	12	11
Black gram, blackeye, mung (av.)	100	**99**	21	45
Broad beans, fresh	120	**71**	28	29
Butter beans, cooked	100	**103**	19	38
Chick peas, cooked	100	**121**	46	37
Green beans, fresh	100	**24**	36	17
Haricot beans, cooked	100	**95**	65	45
Lentils, cooked (all types, average)	100	**105**	22	34
Peas, fresh	100	**83**	21	34
Pinto beans, cooked	100	**137**	47	56
Red kidney beans, cooked	100	**103**	37	45
Runner beans, fresh	100	**22**	33	19
Soya beans, cooked	100	**141**	83	63
Tempeh (fermented soya bean)	100	**166**	120	70
Tofu (soya bean curd)	100	**73**	**1,480**	67

continues

MINERALS			TRACE ELEMENTS					
Phosphorus (mg/portion) (QCT: 550mg/day)	Potassium (mg/portion) (QCT: 2000mg/day)	Sodium Chloride (mg/portion) (max: 3900mg/day)	Copper (mg/portion) (QCT: 1.15mg/day)	Iron (mg/portion) (QCT: 9–12.5mg/day)	Iodine (µg/portion) (QCT: 150µg/day)	Manganese (mg/portion) (QCT: 1.4mg/day)	Selenium (µg/portion) (QCT: 40µg/day)	Zinc (mg/portion) (QCT: 9.4mg/day)
51	380	66	0.02	1.0	n	0.7	tr	0.4
15	170	25	0.02	0.3	2	0.1	1	0.1
63	460	91	0.04	0.8	n	0.1	n	0.3
74	450	10	0.05	0.6	n	0.5	2	0.3
122	1,134	22	0.25	1.3	9	0.4	4	0.9
56	504	121	0.13	0.7	5	0.2	5	0.5
61	468	88	0.11	0.7	9	0.2	2	0.5
112	**1,188**	558	0.25	1.4	9	0.4	4	1.1
40	170	15	0.01	0.1	n	0.1	1	0.3
85	624	68	0.23	1.2	4	0.7	1	0.5
180	570	2	0.51	1.9	n	0.8	2	2.3
124	390	**715**	0.05	1.8	4	0.4	3	0.7
29	44	3	0.05	1.0	n	0.2	n	0.2
140	320	5	0.22	1.9	n	0.5	3	1.1
156	372	1	0.13	1.1	5	0.2	n	1.1
87	400	9	0.16	1.7	n	0.5	n	0.9
83	270	5	0.28	2.1	n	0.7	1	1.2
38	230	tr	0.01	1.2	n	n	n	0.2
120	320	15	0.14	2.5	n	0.7	4	1.0
130	310	3	0.33	3.5	n	0.5	**40**	1.4
130	330	1	0.05	2.8	2	0.4	1	1.1
150	460	1	0.26	2.3	n	0.5	6	1.0
130	420	2	0.23	2.5	n	0.5	6	1.0
34	34	tr	0.02	1.2	2	0.2	n	0.2
250	510	1	0.32	3.0	2	0.7	5	0.9
200	370	6	0.67	**3.6**	n	**1.4**	n	1.8
270	180	12	0.58	3.5	n	1.2	n	2.0

VEGETABLES AND PULSES

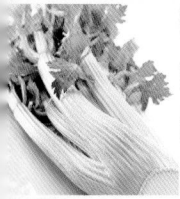

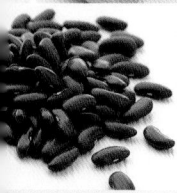

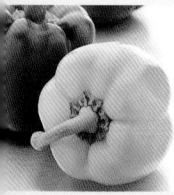

FOOD	AVERAGE PORTION SIZE	TOTAL CALORIES	MINERALS	
(where appropriate, numbers in brackets represent number of vegetables in average portion)	grams per portion	kcals per portion	Calcium (mg/portion) (QCT: 500mg/day)	Magnesium (mg/portion) (QCT: 200mg/day)
Miscellaneous vegetables				
Artichoke hearts (2)	100	**18**	41	23
Asparagus (5 spears)	125	**31**	38	16
Aubergine (1/2)	130	**20**	13	14
Avocado (1)	145	**276**	16	36
Broccoli, green/purple	100	**34**	128	23
Brussels sprouts (9)	100	**42**	26	8
Cabbage (all types, average)	100	**26**	52	8
Cauliflower	100	**34**	21	17
Celery (3 sticks)	100	**7**	41	5
Courgette	100	**18**	25	22
Cucumber (5 cm chunk)	120	**12**	22	10
Curly kale	100	**33**	130	34
Endive	100	**13**	44	10
Fennel	100	**12**	24	8
Lettuce (all types, average)	80	**10**	32	6
Mushrooms, common	100	**13**	6	9
Mushrooms, shiitake	50	**28**	tr	7
Okra	100	**31**	160	71
Olive (10)	30	**31**	18	7
Onion/leek (all types, average)	100	**28**	25	6
Pepper, green/red (1/2)	80	**19**	6	10
Pumpkin	180	**23**	52	18
Seaweed, dried (all types, av.)	10	**8**	66	36
Spinach	100	**25**	170	54
Spring greens	100	**33**	210	19
Sweetcorn	100	**93**	3	37
Swiss chard	100	**19**	51	**81**
Tomato (1)	85	**14**	6	6
Watercress	80	**18**	136	12

MINERALS			TRACE ELEMENTS					
Phosphorus (mg/portion) (QCT: 550mg/day)	Potassium (mg/portion) (QCT: 2000mg/day)	Sodium Chloride (mg/portion) (max: 3900mg/day)	Copper (mg/portion) (QCT: 1.15mg/day)	Iron (mg/portion) (QCT: 9–12.5mg/day)	Iodine (µg/portion) (QCT: 150µg/day)	Manganese (mg/portion) (QCT: 1.4mg/day)	Selenium (µg/portion) (QCT: 40µg/day)	Zinc (mg/portion) (QCT: 9.4mg/day)
38	360	27	0.09	0.7	n	0.3	tr	0.5
90	325	1	0.10	0.5	tr	0.3	1	0.9
21	273	3	0.01	0.4	1	0.1	1	0.3
57	653	9	0.28	0.6	3	0.3	tr	0.6
72	375	9	0.02	1.8	2	0.2	tr	0.6
77	450	6	0.02	0.7	1	0.2	n	0.5
41	270	6	0.02	0.2	2	0.2	1	0.3
64	380	9	0.03	0.7	tr	0.3	tr	0.6
21	320	60	0.02	0.4	n	0.1	3	0.1
45	360	1	0.02	0.8	n	0.1	1	0.3
59	168	4	0.01	0.4	4	0.1	tr	0.1
61	450	43	0.03	1.7	2	0.8	2	0.4
67	380	10	0.01	2.8	n	0.3	1	0.2
26	440	11	0.02	0.3	n	n	n	0.5
28	232	3	0.02	0.9	2	0.2	1	0.2
80	320	5	**0.72**	0.6	3	0.1	9	0.4
15	60	2	n	n	n	n	n	n
59	330	8	0.13	1.1	n	n	1	0.6
5	27	675	0.07	0.3	n	tr	n	n
37	620	4	0.05	1.0	3	0.1	1	0.5
17	112	3	0.02	0.3	1	0.1	tr	0.1
34	234	tr	0.04	0.7	n	0.2	n	0.4
29	117	193	0.12	1.5	**1,683**	0.6	1	**51.0**
45	500	140	0.04	2.1	2	0.6	1	0.7
91	370	20	0.02	3.0	n	n	n	0.4
91	260	1	0.04	0.7	n	0.2	tr	0.4
46	380	210	n	1.8	n	n	n	n
20	213	8	0.09	0.4	2	0.1	tr	0.1
42	184	39	0.01	1.8	n	0.5	n	0.6

VEGETABLE DISHES

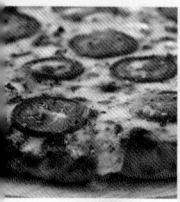

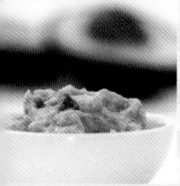

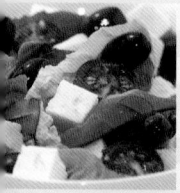

FOOD	AVERAGE PORTION SIZE	TOTAL CALORIES	MINERALS	
(where appropriate, numbers in brackets represent number of items in average portion)	grams per portion	kcals per portion	Calcium (mg/portion) (QCT: 500mg/day)	Magnesium (mg/portion) (QCT: 200mg/day)
Bakes and flans				
Cannelloni	200	**290**	208	28
Casserole, bean and vegetable	250	**115**	58	40
Cauliflower cheese	200	**210**	240	36
Flan, vegetable	120	**253**	145	14
Lasagne, vegetable	450	**527**	329	81
Moussaka, vegetable	350	**480**	266	88
Nut roast	150	**528**	116	**170**
Pizza, cheese and tomato	300	**711**	**630**	57
Shepherd's pie, vegetable	300	**339**	36	42
Burgers, cutlets and pancakes				
Beanburger (no bun)	75	**152**	52	39
Dosa with vegetable filling (1)	200	**307**	48	64
Falafel (3)	100	**179**	80	45
Nut cutlet (2)	120	**347**	101	72
Onion bhaji/pakora (1)	50	**156**	49	31
Pancake with vegetable filling (1)	200	**298**	160	26
Quorn (myco-protein)	100	**86**	28	31
Samosa, vegetable (1)	100	**217**	65	19
Tempeh burger (1)	60	**116**	25	27
Tofu burger (1)	60	**71**	198	26
Vegeburger (1)	60	**147**	54	41
Curries, stews and rice dishes				
Bhaji, cauliflower	250	**535**	68	55
Bhaji, mushroom	250	**415**	45	20
Bhaji, potato	250	**395**	48	60
Broccoli in cheese sauce	200	**236**	320	32
Bubble and squeak	200	**248**	38	18
Curry, cauliflower and potato	250	**148**	53	50
Curry, chick pea and spinach	250	**498**	213	108

continues

MINERALS			TRACE ELEMENTS					
Phosphorus (mg/portion) (QCT: 550mg/day)	Potassium (mg/portion) (QCT: 2000mg/day)	Sodium Chloride (mg/portion) (max: 3900mg/day)	Copper (mg/portion) (QCT: 1.15mg/day)	Iron (mg/portion) (QCT: 9–12.5mg/day)	Iodine (µg/portion) (QCT: 150µg/day)	Manganese (mg/portion) (QCT: 1.4mg/day)	Selenium (µg/portion) (QCT: 40µg/day)	Zinc (mg/portion) (QCT: 9.4mg/day)
186	234	532	0.10	1.0	n	0.4	n	1.2
128	795	322	0.15	1.5	8	0.5	3	0.8
238	618	398	0.06	1.2	22	0.4	2	1.8
110	149	322	0.06	1.0	n	0.2	1	0.7
392	855	**1,755**	0.09	3.6	n	0.9	n	1.8
350	**1,155**	1,575	0.21	3.5	n	0.7	n	1.8
392	632	510	0.81	3.2	14	**2.1**	6	3.0
480	480	1,740	0.36	3.3	**39**	0.9	12	2.4
108	720	1,020	0.21	1.8	n	0.3	**21**	0.9
135	360	165	0.29	1.6	n	0.5	2	1.4
149	600	850	0.32	3.1	8	0.5	2	1.4
130	380	290	0.29	2.8	n	0.5	1	1.0
168	228	252	0.38	1.6	n	0.4	n	1.2
85	275	110	0.16	2.1	2	0.4	1	0.8
166	460	300	0.24	1.6	28	0.3	6	0.8
220	120	310	0.81	0.4	n	**2.1**	n	**7.5**
65	150	390	0.11	1.5	n	0.2	n	0.5
84	108	78	0.23	0.8	n	0.4	n	0.6
102	108	126	0.14	1.1	n	0.6	n	1.0
126	318	252	0.21	2.1	n	0.4	4	0.8
183	1,075	1,050	0.10	2.3	8	0.5	tr	1.8
155	700	n	1.08	1.8	13	0.2	13	1.0
113	975	950	0.25	2.8	13	0.4	3	1.0
260	340	460	0.04	1.4	26	0.1	4	1.4
56	400	14	0.08	0.8	8	0.3	4	0.4
155	1,025	525	0.15	2.0	3	0.5	tr	1.5
218	800	108	0.63	**5.8**	n	1.4	3	2.3

VEGETABLE DISHES

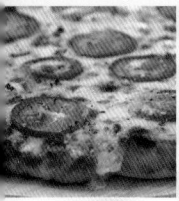

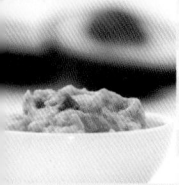

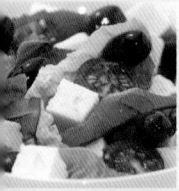

FOOD	AVERAGE PORTION SIZE	TOTAL CALORIES	MINERALS	
(where appropriate, numbers in brackets represent number of items in average portion)	grams per portion	kcals per portion	Calcium (mg/portion) (QCT: 500mg/day)	Magnesium (mg/portion) (QCT: 200mg/day)
Curry, red lentil and mung bean	250	**285**	38	58
Curry, red lentil and tomato	250	**230**	43	40
Curry, okra	250	**273**	300	133
Curry, mixed vegetable	250	**123**	48	28
Okra with tomato and onion	250	**450**	375	165
Ratatouille	250	**205**	43	38
Risotto (brown rice)	350	**501**	88	140
Side dishes, dips, spreads and sauces				
Guacamole	100	**128**	9	19
Houmous	60	**112**	25	37
Laverbread	100	**52**	20	31
Pesto sauce	25	**129**	140	17
Red cabbage, stewed with apple	100	**59**	46	8
Tofu spread	50	**104**	125	9
Vegetable pâté	50	**87**	65	14
Vegetable stir-fry	100	**64**	30	16
Vine leaves, stuffed with rice (3)	100	**262**	130	24
Salads				
Coleslaw, with vinaigrette	100	**87**	37	35
Salad, bean, with vinaigrette	100	**147**	36	24
Salad, beetroot, with vinaigrette	100	**100**	26	14
Salad, carrot, nut, with vinaigrette	100	**218**	38	23
Salad, Greek	100	**130**	61	9
Salad, green (no dressing)	100	**12**	19	7
Salad, pasta, veg., w. mayonnaise	100	**127**	14	11
Salad, potato, with vinaigrette	100	**157**	9	13
Salad, potato, with mayonnaise	100	**239**	8	10
Salad, Waldorf	100	**193**	13	12
Tabouleh orientale	100	**119**	27	33

MINERALS			TRACE ELEMENTS					
Phosphorus (mg/portion) (QCT: 550mg/day)	Potassium (mg/portion) (QCT: 2000mg/day)	Sodium Chloride (mg/portion) (max: 3900mg/day)	Copper (mg/portion) (QCT: 1.15mg/day)	Iron (mg/portion) (QCT: 9–12.5mg/day)	Iodine (µg/portion) (QCT: 150µg/day)	Manganese (mg/portion) (QCT: 1.4mg/day)	Selenium (µg/portion) (QCT: 40µg/day)	Zinc (mg/portion) (QCT: 9.4mg/day)
175	525	525	0.23	4.0	n	n	5	1.5
135	600	525	0.23	3.8	n	n	3	1.3
138	875	750	0.30	2.5	n	n	3	1.3
68	475	53	0.13	2.0	5	0.4	tr	0.5
160	975	325	0.33	3.0	n	n	3	1.5
78	700	500	0.05	1.3	n	0.2	3	0.5
455	910	1,155	**1.30**	4.2	n	1.3	18	2.8
32	370	140	0.13	0.4	2	0.1	tr	0.3
96	114	402	0.18	1.1	n	0.3	n	0.8
51	220	560	0.12	3.5	n	n	n	0.8
120	63	120	0.10	0.6	n	0.3	n	0.9
31	210	32	0.02	0.4	2	0.1	2	0.1
33	60	345	0.06	0.5	n	0.1	n	0.2
95	150	270	0.07	2.1	n	0.2	n	1.1
46	230	11	0.11	0.5	n	0.1	tr	0.3
53	190	1,140	0.56	1.1	4	0.3	2	0.5
24	190	130	0.02	0.4	2	0.1	3	0.2
74	190	280	0.07	1.5	n	0.2	2	0.5
72	420	150	0.03	0.7	n	0.5	tr	0.4
50	300	130	0.18	0.8	3	0.4	1	0.3
61	150	360	0.03	0.4	n	0.1	n	0.2
33	160	6	0.01	0.4	2	0.1	tr	0.1
37	84	51	0.06	0.6	4	0.1	tr	0.4
28	240	120	0.06	0.5	3	0.1	1	0.3
30	210	130	0.05	0.4	12	0.1	n	0.2
35	130	88	0.10	0.3	7	0.2	n	0.3
79	140	76	n	1.8	n	n	n	n

MEAT AND MEAT DISHES

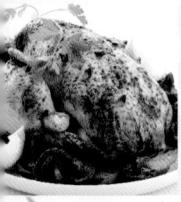

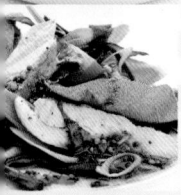

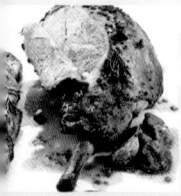

FOOD	AVERAGE PORTION SIZE	TOTAL CALORIES	MINERALS	
	grams per portion	kcals per portion	Calcium (mg/portion) (QCT: 500mg/day)	Magnesium (mg/portion) (QCT: 200mg/day)
Beef				
Mince	200	**458**	36	40
Roast	120	**341**	12	23
Steak	120	**295**	8	29
Veal cutlet	150	**323**	15	50
Lamb				
Chop	160	**443**	11	30
Cutlet	100	**244**	6	15
Roast	120	**319**	10	30
Pork				
Bacon	100	**477**	13	20
Chop	120	**395**	10	20
Roast	120	**343**	12	26
Poultry and game				
Chicken, roast	120	**259**	11	25
Duck, roast	120	**407**	14	19
Goose, roast	120	**383**	12	37
Grouse, roast	120	**208**	36	49
Hare/rabbit, roast or stewed	120	**230**	19	26
Partridge, roast	120	**254**	55	43
Pheasant, roast	120	**256**	59	42
Pigeon, roast	120	**276**	19	43
Turkey, roast	120	**205**	11	29
Venison, roast or stewed	120	**238**	13	26
Offal				
Heart (all types, average)	100	**208**	6	22
Kidney (all types, average)	100	**160**	9	17
Liver (all types, average)	100	**213**	7	20
Oxtail	100	**243**	14	18
Tripe	150	**150**	90	26

continues

MINERALS			TRACE ELEMENTS					
Phosphorus (mg/portion) (QCT: 550mg/day)	Potassium (mg/portion) (QCT: 2000mg/day)	Sodium Chloride (mg/portion) (max: 3900mg/day)	Copper (mg/portion) (QCT: 1.15mg/day)	Iron (mg/portion) (QCT: 9–12.5mg/day)	Iodine (µg/portion) (QCT: 150µg/day)	Manganese (mg/portion) (QCT: 1.4mg/day)	Selenium (µg/portion) (QCT: 40µg/day)	Zinc (mg/portion) (QCT: 9.4mg/day)
340	580	640	0.48	6.2	18	tr	14	**7.8**
204	360	65	0.22	2.3	11	tr	8	4.2
264	432	65	0.18	3.8	13	tr	8	4.2
420	630	165	n	2.0	14	tr	14	4.7
256	400	90	0.21	2.4	11	tr	5	3.2
130	210	47	0.12	1.3	8	tr	3	1.9
240	372	78	0.34	3.0	7	tr	5	6.1
170	300	1,870	0.12	1.3	7	tr	7	1.5
192	348	67	0.16	1.0	10	tr	13	1.6
240	420	95	0.30	1.6	4	tr	24	3.5
204	324	86	0.14	1.0	7	tr	20	2.6
180	252	91	0.32	3.2	n	tr	26	3.1
324	492	180	0.59	5.5	n	tr	n	3.1
408	564	115	n	9.1	n	n	n	n
270	252	43	n	7.6	n	n	19	2.0
372	492	120	n	9.2	n	n	n	n
372	492	120	n	10.1	n	tr	17	1.6
480	492	132	n	**23.3**	n	n	n	n
240	336	62	0.17	1.1	10	tr	20	3.0
348	432	103	n	9.4	n	tr	17	4.7
220	300	105	0.47	4.4	n	tr	n	2.8
250	260	200	0.55	6.0	n	tr	**209**	3.6
350	310	84	**5.08**	11.0	n	0.5	62	5.2
140	170	190	0.27	3.8	n	n	n	8.8
65	180	5	0.21	2.0	n	n	n	n

MEAT AND MEAT DISHES

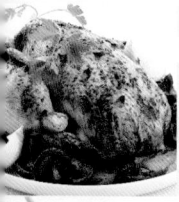

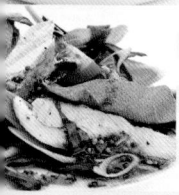

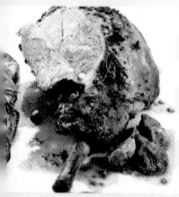

FOOD	AVERAGE PORTION SIZE	TOTAL CALORIES	MINERALS	
(where appropriate, numbers in brackets represent number of items in average portion)	grams per portion	kcals per portion	Calcium (mg/portion) (QCT: 500mg/day)	Magnesium (mg/portion) (QCT: 200mg/day)
Cold meats				
Corned beef	25	**54**	4	4
Ham	25	**30**	tr	5
Luncheon meat	25	**78**	4	2
Tongue	25	**53**	8	4
Burgers and sausages				
Beef burger, quarterpounder	80	**211**	26	18
Liver sausage (1)	50	**155**	13	6
Salami (2 slices)	34	**167**	3	3
Sausage (all types, average) (1)	50	**157**	21	6
Turkey burger/escalope	90	**119**	6	26
Meat dishes				
Black pudding	75	**229**	26	12
Bolognese sauce	220	**306**	57	40
Chicken chow mein	350	**515**	161	39
Cornish pasty	155	**515**	93	28
Haggis	100	**310**	29	36
Hot pot	330	**376**	73	83
Irish stew	330	**409**	40	59
Lamb curry	330	**528**	109	73
Lasagne	350	**669**	**350**	67
Moussaka	330	**644**	290	69
Pork pie	150	**564**	71	24
Samosa (lamb)	100	**578**	35	13
Sausage roll	60	**287**	42	8
Shepherd's pie/cottage pie	300	**357**	45	48
Shish kebab (in pitta with salad)	270	**419**	92	51
Spring roll	100	**242**	32	13
Steak and kidney pie	200	**646**	106	36
Tandoori chicken	350	**749**	203	**126**

MINERALS			TRACE ELEMENTS					
Phosphorus (mg/portion) (QCT: 550mg/day)	Potassium (mg/portion) (QCT: 2000mg/day)	Sodium Chloride (mg/portion) (max: 3900mg/day)	Copper (mg/portion) (QCT: 1.15mg/day)	Iron (mg/portion) (QCT: 9–12.5mg/day)	Iodine (µg/portion) (QCT: 150µg/day)	Manganese (mg/portion) (QCT: 1.4mg/day)	Selenium (µg/portion) (QCT: 40µg/day)	Zinc (mg/portion) (QCT: 9.4mg/day)
30	35	238	0.06	0.7	4	tr	2	1.4
70	70	313	0.06	0.3	1	tr	3	0.5
50	35	263	0.08	0.3	n	tr	2	0.4
35	24	263	0.07	0.6	n	n	n	n
200	272	704	0.20	2.0	5	tr	8	5.0
115	85	430	0.32	3.2	n	0.1	n	1.2
54	54	629	0.08	0.3	5	tr	2	1.0
73	68	425	0.13	0.7	4	0.1	3	0.7
207	306	41	0.13	0.5	n	n	n	1.4
83	105	908	0.28	15.0	n	n	n	1.0
178	682	968	0.31	3.5	15	0.2	9	5.1
224	315	1,631	0.18	3.5	n	0.4	n	0.1
171	295	915	0.54	2.3	5	0.3	3	0.9
160	170	770	0.44	4.8	n	n	n	1.9
274	1,419	**2,211**	0.53	4.0	n	0.3	n	4.3
198	1,122	1,188	0.40	2.0	13	0.3	3	5.0
234	693	1,584	0.53	9.6	23	**0.8**	n	2.0
497	784	1,190	0.32	2.8	**49**	0.4	0	0.6
429	1,155	1,056	0.43	4.3	n	0.4	n	0.3
180	225	1,080	0.48	2.1	11	0.3	9	1.5
n	170	350	0.10	1.0	n	0.5	n	2.3
58	66	330	0.10	0.8	n	n	n	n
207	720	1,350	0.39	3.3	n	n	n	5.7
351	702	891	0.32	4.3	8	0.4	0	0.7
64	117	485	0.06	1.2	n	n	n	0.1
220	280	1,020	0.20	5.0	n	0.3	78	2.4
980	**1,645**	2,065	0.42	6.3	25	0.5	1	0.6

FISH AND FISH DISHES

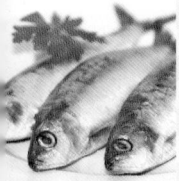

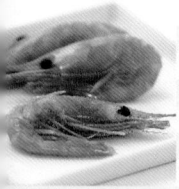

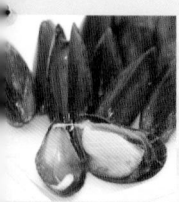

FOOD	AVERAGE PORTION SIZE	TOTAL CALORIES	MINERALS	
	grams per portion	kcals per portion	Calcium (mg/portion) (QCT: 500mg/day)	Magnesium (mg/portion) (QCT: 200mg/day)
White fish				
Cod, fried in batter	120	**239**	80	30
Cod, grilled	120	**114**	12	31
Haddock, fried	120	**209**	144	25
Lemon sole, steamed	120	**109**	25	24
Plaice, fried in batter	120	**308**	88	24
Skate, fried in batter	120	**202**	60	32
Oily fish				
Anchovies, canned	15	**29**	45	8
Herring, grilled	120	**217**	95	**50**
Kipper, grilled	120	**306**	72	37
Mackerel, smoked	150	**531**	30	42
Pilchards, in tomato sauce	50	**72**	125	15
Salmon, canned	50	**77**	46	13
Salmon, grilled	100	**215**	25	32
Salmon, smoked	50	**71**	10	16
Sardines, canned	100	**172**	**540**	45
Trout, grilled	120	**162**	25	31
Tuna, canned	100	**99**	8	27
Seafood				
Lobster, boiled	90	**93**	56	31
Mussels, boiled	40	**42**	21	15
Prawns, boiled	60	**59**	66	29
Shrimps, canned	50	**47**	55	25
Squid, fried in batter	65	**127**	53	15
Fish products and dishes				
Cod roe, fried	120	**242**	16	11
Fish fingers	60	**143**	51	13
Pasta with seafood	250	**275**	95	**50**
Taramasalata	50	**252**	11	3

MINERALS			TRACE ELEMENTS					
Phosphorus (mg/portion) (QCT: 550mg/day)	Potassium (mg/portion) (QCT: 2000mg/day)	Sodium Chloride (mg/portion) (max: 3900mg/day)	Copper (mg/portion) (QCT: 1.15mg/day)	Iron (mg/portion) (QCT: 9–12.5mg/day)	Iodine (µg/portion) (QCT: 150µg/day)	Manganese (mg/portion) (QCT: 1.4mg/day)	Selenium (µg/portion) (QCT: 40µg/day)	Zinc (mg/portion) (QCT: 9.4mg/day)
240	348	192	0.05	0.6	n	0.1	n	0.6
240	456	109	0.05	0.1	156	tr	40	0.6
240	276	348	0.06	1.0	**300**	**0.3**	22	0.5
300	336	144	0.01	0.7	n	n	**88**	0.6
204	252	252	0.07	0.6	n	0.2	7	0.8
216	288	168	0.11	1.2	n	n	n	1.1
45	35	590	0.03	0.6	n	tr	n	0.5
372	**516**	192	0.23	1.9	46	0.1	55	1.4
312	468	**1,128**	0.17	2.2	76	0.1	43	1.3
315	465	1,125	0.14	1.8	150	tr	50	1.7
140	155	145	0.08	1.3	32	0.1	15	0.4
85	130	215	0.03	0.3	30	tr	13	0.4
300	430	54	0.04	0.5	44	tr	31	0.7
125	210	940	0.05	0.3	n	tr	12	0.2
510	320	530	0.16	2.3	23	0.2	41	2.3
300	492	66	0.06	0.5	18	tr	25	0.6
170	230	320	0.05	1.0	13	tr	78	0.7
234	234	297	**1.22**	0.7	90	tr	49	2.3
76	56	144	0.08	**2.7**	48	0.1	17	0.9
162	156	954	0.12	0.7	18	tr	14	1.3
75	50	490	0.12	2.6	41	tr	11	1.0
104	150	57	0.34	0.5	12	0.1	23	0.6
360	204	144	0.26	1.2	n	0.1	n	**4.0**
132	156	270	0.02	0.5	72	0.1	13	0.2
250	475	425	0.18	1.0	98	**0.3**	30	1.3
25	30	325	n	0.2	n	0.1	n	0.2

DAIRY PRODUCTS

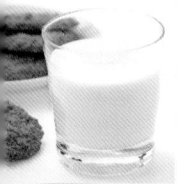

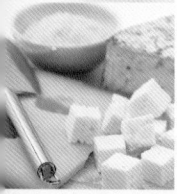

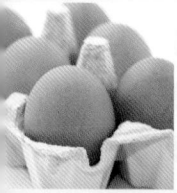

FOOD	AVERAGE PORTION SIZE	TOTAL CALORIES	MINERALS	
	grams/ml per portion	kcals per portion	Calcium (mg/portion) (QCT: 500mg/day)	Magnesium (mg/portion) (QCT: 200mg/day)
Milk				
Skimmed milk	200	**64**	244	22
Semi-skimmed milk	200	**92**	240	22
Whole milk	200	**132**	236	22
Goat's milk	200	**124**	200	26
Soya milk, unsweetened	200	**52**	26	**30**
Milkshake, thick	200	**176**	258	26
Cream				
Single cream	30	**58**	27	2
Double cream	30	**149**	15	2
Crème fraîche	30	**113**	17	2
Cheeses				
Brie/camembert	40	**137**	102	6
Cheddar	40	**166**	296	12
Cottage cheese	40	**40**	51	5
Cream cheese	40	**176**	39	4
Danish blue	40	**137**	195	8
Edam	40	**136**	318	14
Feta	40	**100**	144	8
Goats cheese, soft	40	**128**	53	6
Gouda	40	**151**	309	13
Mozzarella, fresh	40	**103**	145	6
Parmesan, fresh	40	**166**	**410**	16
Stilton	40	**164**	130	6
Yogurt				
Whole-milk yogurt, plain	150	**119**	300	29
Greek-style yogurt, plain	150	**200**	189	20
Greek-style yogurt, sheep's milk	150	**138**	225	24
Soya yogurt, with fruit	150	**110**	21	23
Fromage frais, plain	100	**113**	110	11

continues

MINERALS			TRACE ELEMENTS					
Phosphorus (mg/portion) (QCT: 550mg/day)	Potassium (mg/portion) (QCT: 2000mg/day)	Sodium Chloride (mg/portion) (max: 3900mg/day)	Copper (mg/portion) (QCT: 1.15mg/day)	Iron (mg/portion) (QCT: 9–12.5mg/day)	Iodine (µg/portion) (QCT: 150µg/day)	Manganese (mg/portion) (QCT: 1.4mg/day)	Selenium (µg/portion) (QCT: 40µg/day)	Zinc (mg/portion) (QCT: 9.4mg/day)
192	320	88	tr	0.1	58	tr	2	1.0
188	312	86	tr	tr	60	tr	2	0.8
186	310	86	tr	0.1	62	tr	2	0.8
180	340	84	0.06	0.2	n	tr	n	1.0
96	148	64	0.18	0.9	2	**0.6**	8	0.6
240	342	114	tr	tr	74	tr	4	0.2
24	31	9	tr	tr	n	tr	n	0.1
16	20	7	tr	tr	11	tr	1	0.1
17	24	7	tr	tr	2	tr	0	0.1
93	36	222	tr	tr	6	tr	2	0.8
202	30	289	0.01	0.1	12	tr	2	1.6
68	64	120	tr	tr	10	tr	2	0.2
40	64	120	0.02	tr	n	tr	2	0.2
138	35	488	tr	tr	5	tr	3	1.2
203	36	398	tr	0.1	5	tr	3	1.5
112	38	576	0.03	0.1	n	tr	2	0.4
92	53	240	0.02	tr	20	tr	2	0.4
199	33	370	tr	0.1	n	tr	3	1.6
107	20	158	tr	tr	7	tr	2	1.1
272	61	302	**0.34**	0.3	29	tr	5	**2.0**
126	38	315	0.02	0.1	16	tr	3	1.2
255	**420**	120	tr	0.2	**95**	tr	3	1.1
207	276	99	tr	0.2	59	tr	5	0.8
210	285	225	tr	tr	n	tr	2	0.8
108	141	36	tr	0.8	15	0.3	3	0.3
123	143	36	0.03	0.1	17	tr	3	0.4

DAIRY PRODUCTS

FOOD	AVERAGE PORTION SIZE	TOTAL CALORIES	MINERALS	
	grams per portion	kcals per portion	Calcium (mg/portion) (QCT: 500mg/day)	Magnesium (mg/portion) (QCT: 200mg/day)
Ice cream				
Dairy ice cream	100	**215**	100	12
Non-dairy ice cream	100	**153**	72	11
Eggs and egg dishes				
Egg, boiled	50	**74**	29	6
Egg, fried	60	**107**	39	8
Egg, scrambled	120	**308**	80	14
Omelette	120	**234**	61	14
Quiche	120	**378**	314	22

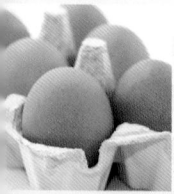

MINERALS			TRACE ELEMENTS					
Phosphorus (mg/portion) (QCT: 550mg/day)	Potassium (mg/portion) (QCT: 2000mg/day)	Sodium Chloride (mg/portion) (max: 3900mg/day)	Copper (mg/portion) (QCT: 1.15mg/day)	Iron (mg/portion) (QCT: 9–12.5mg/day)	Iodine (µg/portion) (QCT: 150µg/day)	Manganese (mg/portion) (QCT: 1.4mg/day)	Selenium (µg/portion) (QCT: 40µg/day)	Zinc (mg/portion) (QCT: 9.4mg/day)
91	174	60	tr	tr	57	tr	2	0.3
74	164	62	tr	0.1	36	tr	2	0.2
100	65	70	0.04	1.0	27	tr	6	0.7
138	90	96	0.05	1.3	36	tr	7	0.9
182	164	266	0.08	1.9	65	tr	11	1.3
210	140	**1,229**	0.08	**2.0**	60	tr	**12**	1.3
272	149	439	0.07	1.2	n	tr	6	1.9

FATS AND OILS

FOOD	AVERAGE PORTION SIZE	TOTAL CALORIES	MINERALS	
(amounts in brackets represent size of average portion)	grams/ml per portion	kcals per portion	Calcium (mg/portion) (QCT: 500mg/day)	Magnesium (mg/portion) (QCT: 200mg/day)
Cooking fats (1tbs)				
Ghee, butter	15	**135**	tr	tr
Ghee, vegetable	15	**134**	tr	tr
Lard	15	**134**	tr	tr
Suet, beef	15	**124**	tr	tr
Suet, vegetable	15	**125**	tr	tr
Table fats (on 1 slice of bread)				
Butter	10	**74**	tr	tr
Spread (eg. Clover)	10	**68**	tr	tr
Low-fat spread (eg. Anchor)	10	**39**	tr	tr
Margarine, hard (eg. Stork)	10	**72**	tr	tr
- hard veg. (eg. Tomor)	10	**74**	tr	tr
- polyunsat. (eg. Blue Band)	10	**75**	tr	tr
Spread (70–80% fat, eg. Flora)	10	**64**	tr	tr
- (60% fat, eg. Vitalite Light)	10	**55**	tr	tr
- with olive oil (eg. Bertolli)	10	**57**	tr	tr
- (35–40% fat, eg. Gold Sunflower)	10	**37**	tr	tr
- (20–25% fat, eg. Outline)	10	**25**	tr	tr
Oils (1 tbs)				
Cod liver oil	15	**135**	tr	tr
Corn oil	15	**135**	tr	tr
Evening primrose oil	15	**135**	tr	tr
Grapeseed oil	15	**135**	tr	tr
Olive oil	15	**135**	tr	tr
Safflower oil	15	**135**	tr	tr
Sesame oil	15	**135**	tr	tr
Sunflower oil	15	**135**	tr	tr
Vegetable oil, blended	15	**135**	tr	tr
Walnut oil	15	**135**	tr	tr
Wheat germ oil	15	**135**	tr	tr

MINERALS			TRACE ELEMENTS					
Phosphorus (mg/portion) (QCT: 550mg/day)	Potassium (mg/portion) (QCT: 2000mg/day)	Sodium Chloride (mg/portion) (max: 3900mg/day)	Copper (mg/portion) (QCT: 1.15mg/day)	Iron (mg/portion) (QCT: 9–12.5mg/day)	Iodine (µg/portion) (QCT: 150µg/day)	Manganese (mg/portion) (QCT: 1.4mg/day)	Selenium (µg/portion) (QCT: 40µg/day)	Zinc (mg/portion) (QCT: 9.4mg/day)
tr	tr	tr	tr	tr	n	tr	tr	tr
tr	tr	tr	**0.02**	tr	n	tr	tr	tr
tr	tr	tr	tr	tr	tr	tr	tr	tr
tr	tr	tr	tr	tr	1	tr	tr	tr
tr	tr	2	tr	tr	tr	tr	tr	tr
tr	tr	75	tr	tr	**4**	tr	tr	tr
tr	tr	67	tr	tr	n	tr	tr	tr
tr	tr	51	tr	tr	n	tr	tr	tr
tr	tr	**94**	tr	tr	n	tr	n	n
tr	tr	40	tr	tr	n	tr	n	n
tr	tr	68	tr	tr	n	tr	n	n
tr	tr	80	tr	tr	n	tr	n	n
tr	tr	71	tr	tr	n	tr	n	n
tr	tr	60	tr	tr	n	tr	n	n
tr	tr	65	tr	tr	n	tr	n	n
tr	tr	54	tr	tr	n	tr	n	n
tr	tr	tr	tr	tr	tr	tr	tr	tr
tr	tr	tr	tr	tr	tr	tr	tr	tr
tr	tr	tr	tr	tr	tr	tr	tr	tr
tr	tr	tr	tr	tr	tr	tr	tr	tr
tr	tr	tr	tr	tr	tr	tr	tr	tr
tr	tr	tr	tr	tr	tr	tr	tr	tr
tr	tr	tr	tr	tr	tr	tr	tr	tr
tr	tr	tr	tr	tr	tr	tr	tr	tr
tr	tr	tr	tr	tr	tr	tr	tr	tr
tr	tr	tr	tr	tr	tr	tr	tr	tr
tr	tr	tr	tr	tr	tr	tr	tr	tr

GRAINS, CEREALS, BREADS

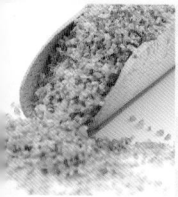

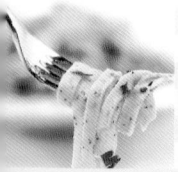

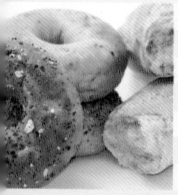

FOOD	AVERAGE PORTION SIZE	TOTAL CALORIES	MINERALS	
	grams per portion	kcals per portion	Calcium (mg/portion) (QCT: 500mg/day)	Magnesium (mg/portion) (QCT: 200mg/day)
Flours and grains				
Barley, pearl	100	**360**	20	65
Buckwheat	100	**364**	12	48
Bulgur wheat	100	**353**	44	140
Cornflour	100	**354**	15	7
Couscous	100	**227**	19	n
Custard powder	100	**354**	15	7
Millet	100	**354**	55	110
Oatmeal	100	**401**	55	110
Quinoa	100	**309**	79	210
Rice, brown	200	**282**	8	86
Rice, white	200	**276**	36	22
Rice flour	100	**366**	24	23
Rye flour	100	**335**	32	92
Soya flour	100	**447**	210	**240**
Wheat flour, white	100	**341**	140	20
Wheat flour, wholemeal	100	**310**	38	120
Wheat germ	25	**76**	14	30
Wheat bran	15	**31**	17	78
Noodles and pasta (cooked)				
Noodles, egg	300	**186**	15	24
Noodles, plain	300	**186**	15	24
Pasta, white	300	**312**	21	45
Pasta, wholemeal	300	**339**	33	126
Pastry				
Puff pastry	100	**373**	58	12
Shortcrust pastry	100	**449**	85	15
Breakfast cereals				
All-bran	50	**126**	35	185
Coco pops	50	**193**	18	n

continues

MINERALS			TRACE ELEMENTS					
Phosphorus (mg/portion) (QCT: 550mg/day)	Potassium (mg/portion) (QCT: 2000mg/day)	Sodium Chloride (mg/portion) (max: 3900mg/day)	Copper (mg/portion) (QCT: 1.15mg/day)	Iron (mg/portion) (QCT: 9–12.5mg/day)	Iodine (µg/portion) (QCT: 150µg/day)	Manganese (mg/portion) (QCT: 1.4mg/day)	Selenium (µg/portion) (QCT: 40µg/day)	Zinc (mg/portion) (QCT: 9.4mg/day)
210	270	3	0.40	3.0	n	1.3	1	2.1
150	220	1	0.70	2.0	n	1.6	**9**	2.6
330	290	5	0.56	4.9	n	n	n	n
39	61	52	0.13	1.4	n	n	n	0.3
240	n	n	n	5.0	n	n	n	n
39	61	320	0.05	1.4	n	n	n	0.3
380	370	33	0.23	4.1	n	3.7	3	3.3
380	370	33	0.23	4.1	n	**3.9**	3	3.3
230	780	61	0.82	**7.8**	n	n	n	3.3
240	198	2	0.66	1.0	n	1.8	8	1.4
108	108	2	0.26	0.4	7	0.4	8	1.4
130	240	5	0.20	1.9	n	n	n	n
360	410	1	0.42	2.7	n	0.7	n	3.0
600	**1,660**	9	**2.92**	6.9	n	2.3	**9**	3.9
110	150	3	0.15	2.0	7	0.6	4	0.6
320	340	3	0.45	3.9	n	3.1	6	2.9
263	238	1	0.23	2.1	n	3.1	1	**4.3**
180	174	4	0.20	1.9	n	1.4	tr	2.4
93	69	45	0.18	0.9	n	0.5	n	0.9
84	39	3	0.18	0.9	tr	0.5	tr	0.9
132	72	tr	0.30	1.5	tr	0.8	tr	1.5
330	420	135	0.54	4.2	n	2.7	n	3.3
54	70	310	0.14	0.9	n	0.2	n	0.4
68	91	410	0.10	1.3	7	0.4	2	0.4
310	450	**740**	0.22	6.0	n	n	n	4.2
60	95	440	0.10	3.4	n	n	n	n

GRAINS, CEREALS, BREADS

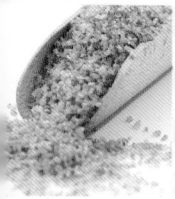

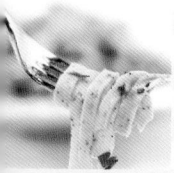

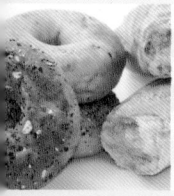

FOOD	AVERAGE PORTION SIZE	TOTAL CALORIES	MINERALS	
(where appropriate, numbers in brackets represent number of items in average portion)	grams per portion	kcals per portion	Calcium (mg/portion) (QCT: 500mg/day)	Magnesium (mg/portion) (QCT: 200mg/day)
Corn flakes	50	**178**	8	7
Fruit 'n' Fibre	50	**176**	26	n
Grapenuts	50	**173**	19	48
Muesli (Swiss style)	70	**255**	84	60
Porridge (made with water)	200	**98**	14	36
Puffed wheat	50	**161**	13	70
Rice Krispies	50	**185**	10	25
Shredded wheat (2)	50	**163**	19	65
Special K	50	**190**	35	26
Weetabix (2)	40	**142**	14	48
Breads and rolls				
Bagel (1)	90	**246**	5	31
Brown bread (1 slice)	40	**87**	40	21
Chapati (1)	55	**111**	33	20
French baguette (5 cm slice)	40	**108**	52	24
Granary bread (1 slice)	40	**94**	31	45
Naan bread (1)	160	**538**	**256**	44
Papadum (fried) (2)	26	**96**	18	23
Pitta bread (1 large)	95	**252**	86	12
Rye bread (1 slice)	25	**55**	20	22
Wheat germ bread (1 slice)	40	**105**	48	10
White bread (1 slice)	40	**94**	44	11
Wholemeal bread (1 slice)	40	**86**	22	30
Croissant (1)	50	**180**	40	13
Hamburger bun (1)	50	**132**	65	16
Morning roll (1)	50	**135**	70	17
Wholemeal roll (1)	50	**121**	28	35

MINERALS			TRACE ELEMENTS					
Phosphorus (mg/portion) (QCT: 550mg/day)	Potassium (mg/portion) (QCT: 2000mg/day)	Sodium Chloride (mg/portion) (max: 3900mg/day)	Copper (mg/portion) (QCT: 1.15mg/day)	Iron (mg/portion) (QCT: 9–12.5mg/day)	Iodine (µg/portion) (QCT: 150µg/day)	Manganese (mg/portion) (QCT: 1.4mg/day)	Selenium (µg/portion) (QCT: 40µg/day)	Zinc (mg/portion) (QCT: 9.4mg/day)
19	50	555	0.02	3.4	3	tr	1	0.2
100	225	280	0.12	3.4	n	n	n	n
125	155	295	0.23	4.8	n	n	n	2.1
196	308	266	0.07	3.9	n	n	n	1.8
94	92	66	0.06	1.0	n	0.9	n	0.8
175	195	2	0.28	2.3	n	n	n	1.4
65	75	630	0.05	3.4	n	0.5	n	0.6
170	165	4	0.20	2.1	n	n	n	1.2
120	115	575	0.07	6.7	n	n	n	1.0
116	148	148	0.22	2.4	n	n	n	0.8
25	360	1	0.09	0.3	7	0.4	1	0.2
60	68	216	0.06	0.9	n	0.5	n	0.4
66	83	66	0.11	1.2	n	0.7	n	0.6
44	52	228	0.06	0.8	2	0.2	2	0.3
72	76	232	0.07	1.1	n	0.6	n	0.6
208	288	608	0.19	2.1	**20**	0.7	tr	1.3
65	195	637	0.13	2.9	n	0.3	n	0.7
87	105	494	0.20	1.6	n	0.4	n	0.6
40	48	145	0.05	0.6	n	0.3	n	0.3
72	76	228	0.08	1.2	6	0.7	n	0.8
36	44	208	0.08	0.6	2	0.2	2	0.2
80	92	220	0.10	1.1	tr	0.8	3	0.7
65	70	195	0.13	1.0	n	0.2	n	0.5
75	55	275	0.07	1.2	6	0.2	5	0.4
60	65	320	0.10	1.1	6	0.3	3	0.5
85	115	230	0.13	1.8	tr	0.8	4	0.8

BISCUITS, CAKES, PUDDINGS

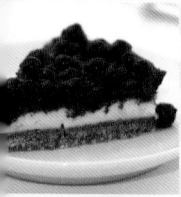

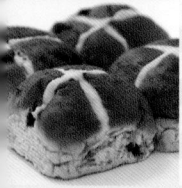

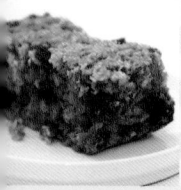

FOOD	AVERAGE PORTION SIZE	TOTAL CALORIES	MINERALS	
(where appropriate, numbers in brackets represent number of items in average portion)	grams per portion	kcals per portion	Calcium (mg/portion) (QCT: 500mg/day)	Magnesium (mg/portion) (QCT: 200mg/day)
Biscuits				
Chocolate biscuit (1)	25	**131**	28	11
Cream cracker (1)	15	**66**	17	4
Crispbread, rye (1)	10	**32**	5	10
Digestive biscuit, plain (1)	15	**71**	14	3
Flapjack (1)	60	**290**	22	29
Wholemeal biscuit (1)	15	**54**	17	18
Oatcake (1)	15	**66**	8	15
Rich tea/Marie biscuits (1)	10	**46**	12	2
Shortbread (1)	15	**75**	14	2
Water biscuit (1)	10	**44**	12	2
Wholemeal cracker (1)	15	**62**	17	7
Cakes				
Chocolate cake (1 slice)	70	**319**	53	**32**
Fruit cake (1 slice)	70	**248**	42	18
Gâteau (1 slice)	70	**236**	42	6
Sponge cake (1 slice)	70	**321**	46	6
Swiss roll (1 slice)	35	**97**	34	4
Puddings				
Cheesecake (1 slice)	110	**452**	70	10
Christmas pudding	100	**291**	79	27
Fruit crumble	170	**337**	83	15
Custard (made with milk)	150	**176**	**195**	20
Fruit pie	120	**223**	58	11
Pancake (1)	110	**331**	121	15
Rice pudding	200	**178**	186	22
Trifle	170	**272**	134	26
Buns and pastries				
Crumpet (1)	40	**71**	44	6
Currant bun (1)	60	**178**	66	16

continues

MINERALS			TRACE ELEMENTS					
Phosphorus (mg/portion) (QCT: 550mg/day)	Potassium (mg/portion) (QCT: 2000mg/day)	Sodium Chloride (mg/portion) (max: 3900mg/day)	Copper (mg/portion) (QCT: 1.15mg/day)	Iron (mg/portion) (QCT: 9–12.5mg/day)	Iodine (µg/portion) (QCT: 150µg/day)	Manganese (mg/portion) (QCT: 1.4mg/day)	Selenium (µg/portion) (QCT: 40µg/day)	Zinc (mg/portion) (QCT: 9.4mg/day)
33	58	40	0.06	0.4	n	n	n	0.2
17	18	92	0.03	0.3	2	0.1	1	0.1
31	50	22	0.04	0.4	2	0.4	tr	0.3
13	26	90	0.04	0.5	n	0.1	n	0.1
96	120	168	0.14	1.3	n	**1.2**	1	**0.9**
51	59	71	0.06	0.5	n	0.4	7	0.4
63	51	185	0.06	0.7	n	0.5	n	0.3
8	14	41	0.01	0.2	n	n	n	0.1
11	15	35	0.02	0.2	3	0.1	tr	0.1
9	14	47	0.01	0.2	n	n	n	0.1
26	30	105	0.04	0.4	n	0.2	n	0.2
147	133	301	**0.27**	1.3	24	0.1	4	0.8
77	273	175	0.18	1.2	**105**	n	n	0.4
66	62	39	0.04	0.6	12	0.1	n	0.4
105	57	245	0.07	0.8	18	0.1	4	0.5
63	39	46	0.04	0.5	9	n	3	0.2
105	121	341	0.12	1.0	n	0.1	n	0.7
76	350	200	0.22	1.5	n	0.4	7	0.5
56	323	116	0.17	1.0	10	0.3	2	0.3
165	255	122	tr	0.2	n	n	n	0.6
40	216	144	0.12	0.6	6	0.2	1	0.2
121	165	58	0.06	0.9	26	0.2	3	0.7
160	280	100	0.06	0.4	n	n	n	0.8
145	255	92	0.07	1.0	n	0.1	n	0.7
64	33	288	0.07	0.4	0	0.1	10	0.2
60	126	138	0.11	1.1	n	0.3	n	0.4

BISCUITS, CAKES, PUDDINGS

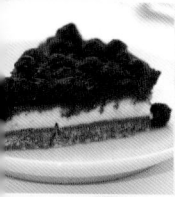

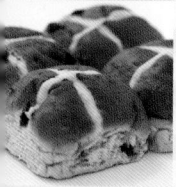

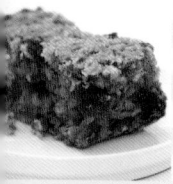

FOOD	AVERAGE PORTION SIZE	TOTAL CALORIES	MINERALS	
(where appropriate, numbers in brackets represent number of items in average portion)	grams per portion	kcals per portion	Calcium (mg/portion) (QCT: 500mg/day)	Magnesium (mg/portion) (QCT: 200mg/day)
Danish pastry (1)	110	**411**	101	26
Doughnut (jam) (1)	75	**252**	54	14
Greek pastry (Baklava) (1)	100	**322**	44	22
Hot cross bun (1)	50	**155**	55	12
Jam tart (1)	25	**95**	14	3
Mince pie (1)	50	**212**	38	8
Muffin (American)	70	**256**	39	25
Muffin (English) (1)	70	**198**	98	20
Scone (1)	50	**181**	90	9
Teacake (1)	60	**178**	53	17
Waffle (1)	65	**217**	169	14

MINERALS			TRACE ELEMENTS					
Phosphorus (mg/portion) (QCT: 550mg/day)	Potassium (mg/portion) (QCT: 2000mg/day)	Sodium Chloride (mg/portion) (max: 3900mg/day)	Copper (mg/portion) (QCT: 1.15mg/day)	Iron (mg/portion) (QCT: 9–12.5mg/day)	Iodine (µg/portion) (QCT: 150µg/day)	Manganese (mg/portion) (QCT: 1.4mg/day)	Selenium (µg/portion) (QCT: 40µg/day)	Zinc (mg/portion) (QCT: 9.4mg/day)
108	187	209	0.07	1.4	n	0.4	n	0.6
53	83	135	0.07	0.9	18	0.2	n	0.4
70	90	310	0.14	0.9	n	0.3	n	0.4
55	100	60	0.12	0.8	n	0.2	n	0.4
12	28	58	0.04	0.4	3	n	tr	0.1
29	90	155	0.08	0.8	n	0.2	n	0.2
46	**525**	11	0.21	0.7	4	0.1	1	0.4
105	126	91	0.14	1.3	n	0.3	**20**	0.6
230	75	**385**	0.10	0.7	10	0.2	1	0.4
60	132	162	0.14	**1.6**	n	0.3	n	0.4
241	124	377	0.07	0.9	22	0.2	3	0.5

SUGAR PRODUCTS

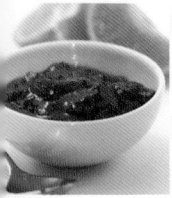

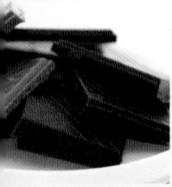

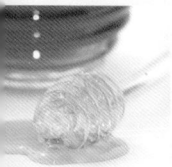

FOOD	AVERAGE PORTION SIZE	TOTAL CALORIES	MINERALS	
(where appropriate, numbers in brackets represent size of average portion)	grams per portion	kcals per portion	Calcium (mg/portion) (QCT: 500mg/day)	Magnesium (mg/portion) (QCT: 200mg/day)
Sugars and syrups (1 tbs)				
Honey	20	**58**	tr	tr
Molasses	20	**53**	42	48
Sugar, brown	20	**72**	11	3
Sugar, white	20	**79**	tr	tr
Syrup, golden	20	**60**	3	tr
Syrup, maple	20	**52**	13	3
Treacle, black	20	**51**	110	36
Preserves and spreads (1 tbs)				
Chocolate nut spread	20	**110**	9	10
Fruit spread	20	**24**	5	6
Jam	20	**52**	16	9
Marmalade	20	**52**	17	12
Chocolate				
Chocolate bar (eg. Mars, Twix)	50	**221**	80	18
Milk chocolate	50	**260**	110	25
Plain chocolate	50	**255**	17	45
Confectionery				
Boiled sweets	50	**164**	3	1
Cereal crunchy bar	50	**234**	39	43
Fruit pastilles	50	**164**	14	3
Halva (with carrot)	50	**177**	75	10
Liquorice shapes	50	**139**	**220**	**85**
Nougat	50	**192**	13	12
Peppermints	50	**197**	4	2
Turkish delight (with nuts)	50	**172**	11	4

MINERALS			TRACE ELEMENTS					
Phosphorus (mg/portion) (QCT: 550mg/day)	Potassium (mg/portion) (QCT: 2000mg/day)	Sodium Chloride (mg/portion) (max: 3900mg/day)	Copper (mg/portion) (QCT: 1.15mg/day)	Iron (mg/portion) (QCT: 9–12.5mg/day)	Iodine (µg/portion) (QCT: 150µg/day)	Manganese (mg/portion) (QCT: 1.4mg/day)	Selenium (µg/portion) (QCT: 40µg/day)	Zinc (mg/portion) (QCT: 9.4mg/day)
3	10	2	0.01	0.1	tr	0.1	tr	0.2
6	292	7	0.10	0.9	tr	0.3	tr	0.1
tr	28	6	0.01	0.3	tr	tr	tr	tr
tr	tr	1	0.02	tr	tr	tr	tr	tr
tr	12	54	0.01	0.1	tr	tr	tr	tr
tr	40	2	0.01	0.2	tr	0.7	tr	0.8
6	352	36	0.16	4.3	tr	0.5	n	0.2
36	96	44	0.08	0.4	n	0.2	tr	0.4
15	60	85	0.03	0.3	1	0.1	tr	0.1
26	76	58	0.06	0.6	n	0.1	tr	0.2
28	38	42	0.06	0.3	n	0.1	n	0.2
75	125	75	0.16	0.6	n	0.2	1	0.6
110	195	43	0.12	0.7	**15**	0.1	**2**	0.6
70	150	3	**0.36**	1.2	2	0.3	**2**	0.7
6	tr	13	0.05	0.2	n	n	tr	n
145	180	37	0.15	1.3	n	1.1	n	**0.9**
tr	14	17	0.02	0.2	n	tr	tr	tr
65	185	50	0.04	0.3	9	0.1	1	0.3
37	**795**	**95**	**0.36**	**8.4**	n	**1.3**	n	0.5
37	120	60	0.11	0.4	n	0.1	1	0.3
tr	tr	5	0.02	0.1	n	n	tr	n
11	27	42	0.07	0.2	tr	tr	1	0.1

SOUPS AND SAUCES

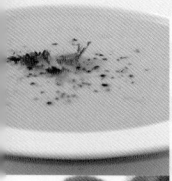

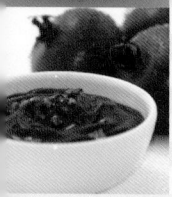

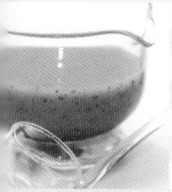

FOOD	AVERAGE PORTION SIZE	TOTAL CALORIES	MINERALS	
	grams/ml per portion	kcals per portion	Calcium (mg/portion) (QCT: 500mg/day)	Magnesium (mg/portion) (QCT: 200mg/day)
Soups				
Bouillabaisse	250	**338**	**113**	**35**
Carrot and orange soup	250	**50**	33	5
Chicken soup	250	**145**	68	13
French onion soup	250	**100**	8	5
Gazpacho	250	**113**	28	20
Leek and potato soup	250	**130**	73	18
Lentil soup	250	**293**	40	50
Minestrone soup	250	**158**	35	18
Mushroom soup	250	**115**	75	10
Oxtail soup	250	**110**	100	15
Tomato soup	250	**130**	43	20
Vegetable soup	250	**130**	33	10
Sauces				
Black bean sauce	30	**28**	26	14
Brown sauce (spicy)	30	**36**	11	16
Curry sauce	115	**90**	35	21
Dressing, French	30	**139**	n	n
Dressing, Thousand Island	30	**97**	7	3
Dressing, yogurt-based	30	**88**	17	2
Gravy (instant)	70	**24**	tr	tr
Hollandaise sauce	70	**495**	39	6
Mayonnaise	30	**207**	tr	tr
Mint sauce	10	**10**	12	5
Raita	50	**29**	75	9
Salad cream	30	**104**	5	3
Soy sauce	10	**4**	tr	4
Sweet and sour sauce	150	**66**	15	9
Tomato ketchup	30	**35**	4	6

MINERALS			TRACE ELEMENTS					
Phosphorus (mg/portion) (QCT: 550mg/day)	Potassium (mg/portion) (QCT: 2000mg/day)	Sodium Chloride (mg/portion) (max: 3900mg/day)	Copper (mg/portion) (QCT: 1.15mg/day)	Iron (mg/portion) (QCT: 9–12.5mg/day)	Iodine (µg/portion) (QCT: 150µg/day)	Manganese (mg/portion) (QCT: 1.4mg/day)	Selenium (µg/portion) (QCT: 40µg/day)	Zinc (mg/portion) (QCT: 9.4mg/day)
400	**525**	135	0.13	1.8	n	0.1	n	1.0
25	213	375	0.03	0.5	3	0.1	tr	0.3
68	103	1,000	0.05	1.0	5	tr	tr	0.8
10	135	198	0.03	0.3	tr	tr	tr	tr
53	450	325	0.10	0.8	n	n	tr	0.3
88	400	208	0.05	1.0	10	0.2	3	0.5
200	**525**	225	**0.50**	**4.5**	n	n	n	**1.8**
70	300	350	0.13	1.3	n	**0.3**	n	0.5
75	138	**1,175**	0.10	0.8	8	tr	3	0.8
93	233	1,100	0.10	2.5	3	tr	tr	1.0
50	475	1,000	0.15	1.0	8	**0.3**	tr	0.5
50	275	325	0.05	0.8	n	0.2	3	0.3
25	45	753	0.06	1.7	n	0.2	n	0.2
6	99	450	0.03	0.4	n	0.1	n	0.1
36	207	1,127	0.06	1.3	n	0.2	n	0.2
n	n	138	n	n	n	n	n	n
10	39	270	0.02	0.1	2	tr	tr	0.1
18	36	195	tr	tr	n	tr	n	0.1
tr	tr	322	0.01	tr	n	tr	n	tr
105	44	700	0.06	1.6	**48**	0.1	**4**	0.8
8	tr	135	0.01	0.1	11	tr	n	tr
tr	21	69	0.03	0.7	tr	0.1	tr	tr
65	125	175	tr	0.1	22	0.1	tr	0.3
14	12	312	tr	0.2	3	tr	n	0.1
5	18	712	tr	0.2	n	tr	n	tr
15	140	585	0.03	0.8	n	**0.3**	n	0.2
9	105	489	0.02	0.1	n	tr	n	tr

PICKLES AND SAVOURIES

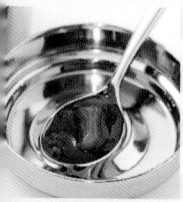

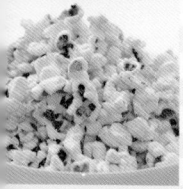

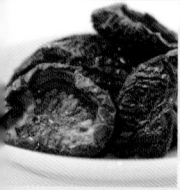

FOOD	AVERAGE PORTION SIZE	TOTAL CALORIES	MINERALS	
(where appropriate, numbers in brackets represent number of items in average portion)	grams per portion	kcals per portion	Calcium (mg/portion) (QCT: 500mg/day)	Magnesium (mg/portion) (QCT: 200mg/day)
Pickles and chutneys				
Lime pickle	40	**71**	48	32
Piccalilli	40	**34**	6	2
Relish (corn/cucumber/onion)	40	**48**	5	4
Sweet mango chutney	40	**76**	4	8
Tomato chutney	40	**51**	9	5
Tomatoes, sun-dried	50	**248**	16	14
Savoury snacks				
Bombay mix	30	**164**	23	42
Breadsticks (3)	20	**78**	5	5
Popcorn, plain	50	**297**	5	41
Pork scratchings	25	**152**	8	5
Potato crisps	40	**212**	12	16
Potato crisps, low-fat	40	**183**	14	19
Pretzels	50	**191**	18	18
Tortilla chips	50	**230**	**75**	**45**
Twiglets	50	**192**	23	41

MINERALS			TRACE ELEMENTS					
Phosphorus (mg/portion) (QCT: 550mg/day)	Potassium (mg/portion) (QCT: 2000mg/day)	Sodium Chloride (mg/portion) (max: 3900mg/day)	Copper (mg/portion) (QCT: 1.15mg/day)	Iron (mg/portion) (QCT: 9–12.5mg/day)	Iodine (µg/portion) (QCT: 150µg/day)	Manganese (mg/portion) (QCT: 1.4mg/day)	Selenium (µg/portion) (QCT: 40µg/day)	Zinc (mg/portion) (QCT: 9.4mg/day)
n	96	212	0.08	**2.3**	n	n	n	0.1
7	16	536	0.01	0.2	n	tr	n	tr
10	44	136	0.03	0.1	n	tr	n	0.1
3	17	520	tr	0.4	n	tr	n	tr
13	116	52	0.04	0.4	1	0.1	tr	0.1
23	230	500	**0.41**	1.0	**24**	0.1	tr	0.4
120	156	249	0.30	0.8	n	0.5	n	**1.4**
22	32	172	0.02	0.2	n	0.1	n	0.1
85	110	2	n	0.6	1	0.2	n	0.9
45	75	330	0.05	0.6	n	tr	n	0.4
44	376	336	0	0.6	n	0.1	n	0.2
52	**408**	292	0.15	0.7	n	0.2	n	0.4
55	75	**860**	0.13	2.2	n	**0.9**	n	0.5
120	110	430	0.05	0.8	n	0.2	n	0.6
185	230	670	0.16	1.5	n	0.8	n	1.0

DRINKS

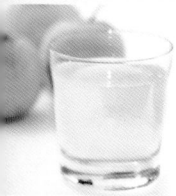

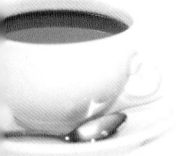

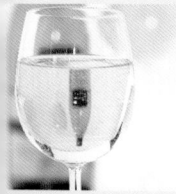

FOOD	AVERAGE PORTION SIZE	TOTAL CALORIES	MINERALS	
(where appropriate, numbers in brackets represent size of average portion)	ml per portion	kcals per portion	Calcium (mg/portion) (QCT: 500mg/day)	Magnesium (mg/portion) (QCT: 200mg/day)
Fruit juices (unsweetened)				
Apple juice	200	**76**	14	10
Cranberry juice	200	**122**	**110**	**70**
Grape juice	200	**92**	38	14
Grapefruit juice	200	**66**	28	16
Lemon juice	20	**1**	tr	1
Lime juice	20	**2**	tr	1
Mango juice (canned)	200	**78**	4	n
Orange juice	200	**66**	24	24
Passion fruit juice	200	**94**	14	58
Pineapple juice	200	**82**	16	12
Pomegranate juice	200	**88**	6	6
Prune juice	200	**114**	28	22
Hot drinks				
Coffee, black	190	**4**	6	15
Coffee, with milk	190	**13**	29	15
Coffee, Irish	190	**160**	21	11
Drinking chocolate (for 1 mug)	18	**66**	6	27
Horlicks (for 1 mug)	24	**95**	55	11
Ovaltine (for 1 mug)	24	**91**	9	36
Tea, black	190	**tr**	tr	4
Tea, with milk	190	**15**	25	6
Tea, green	190	**tr**	4	tr
Tea, herbal	190	**2**	4	2
Soft drinks (carbonated)				
Cola	330	**129**	20	3
Fruit juice drink (eg. Tango)	330	**129**	23	23
Ginger ale	250	**38**	n	n
Lemonade	200	**44**	10	2

continues

MINERALS			TRACE ELEMENTS					
Phosphorus (mg/portion) (QCT: 550mg/day)	Potassium (mg/portion) (QCT: 2000mg/day)	Sodium Chloride (mg/portion) (max: 3900mg/day)	Copper (mg/portion) (QCT: 1.15mg/day)	Iron (mg/portion) (QCT: 9–12.5mg/day)	Iodine (µg/portion) (QCT: 150µg/day)	Manganese (mg/portion) (QCT: 1.4mg/day)	Selenium (µg/portion) (QCT: 40µg/day)	Zinc (mg/portion) (QCT: 9.4mg/day)
12	220	4	tr	0.2	tr	tr	tr	tr
130	**1,500**	30	**0.60**	2.0	**10**	0.4	**4**	1.0
28	110	14	tr	1.8	n	0.2	2	0.2
22	200	14	0.02	0.4	n	0.4	2	tr
tr	26	tr	0.01	tr	n	tr	0	tr
tr	22	tr	0.01	tr	n	tr	n	0
44	36	18	n	**3.0**	n	n	n	n
44	360	4	tr	0.6	4	0.2	2	tr
42	400	38	n	1.0	n	n	n	**1.6**
tr	106	16	0.04	0.4	tr	**1.4**	tr	0.2
16	400	2	0.14	0.4	n	n	n	n
38	420	24	0.08	1.4	6	0.2	tr	0.4
13	175	tr	tr	0.2	tr	0.1	tr	tr
30	184	11	tr	0.2	4	0.1	tr	0.2
25	137	11	tr	0.2	tr	0.1	tr	0.2
34	74	45	0.20	0.4	n	n	n	0.3
72	180	**84**	0.19	0.4	n	n	n	n
96	204	36	0.29	0.6	n	n	n	n
4	51	tr	0.02	tr	tr	0.3	tr	tr
23	76	11	0.02	0	n	0.3	tr	0.2
tr	38	2	tr	0.2	tr	tr	tr	tr
tr	17	tr	0.04	0.2	tr	0.1	tr	tr
99	3	17	tr	tr	tr	tr	tr	tr
7	89	26	tr	tr	tr	tr	tr	tr
n	n	n	n	n	tr	tr	tr	n
tr	30	14	tr	tr	tr	tr	tr	tr

DRINKS

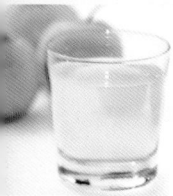

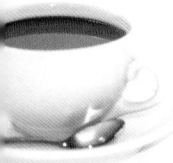

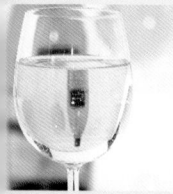

FOOD	AVERAGE PORTION SIZE	TOTAL CALORIES	MINERALS	
	ml per portion	kcals per portion	Calcium (mg/portion) (QCT: 500mg/day)	Magnesium (mg/portion) (QCT: 200mg/day)
Lucozade	200	**120**	14	14
Tonic water	250	**83**	3	0
Soft drinks (uncarbonated)				
Barley water (diluted)	200	**28**	tr	tr
Ribena (diluted)	200	**60**	tr	tr
Fruit juice drink (diluted)	200	**74**	12	6
Rosehip syrup (diluted)	200	**92**	n	n
Alcoholic drinks				
Beer, bitter	300	**177**	24	21
Beer, lager	300	**384**	15	21
Beer, shandy	300	**48**	24	3
Beer, stout	300	**156**	12	24
Cider	300	**108**	24	9
Champagne	125	**95**	4	8
Red wine	125	**85**	9	14
White wine	125	**83**	11	10
Port	50	**79**	tr	6
Sherry	50	**58**	4	7
Vermouth/martini	50	**55**	4	3
Cream liqueurs (eg. Baileys)	25	**81**	5	tr
Liqueurs, high-strength (eg. pernod)	25	**79**	tr	tr
Liqueurs, med.-strength (eg. campari)	25	**66**	tr	tr
Spirits (eg. brandy/gin/whisky)	25	**56**	tr	tr

MINERALS			TRACE ELEMENTS					
Phosphorus (mg/portion) (QCT: 550mg/day)	Potassium (mg/portion) (QCT: 2000mg/day)	Sodium Chloride (mg/portion) (max: 3900mg/day)	Copper (mg/portion) (QCT: 1.15mg/day)	Iron (mg/portion) (QCT: 9–12.5mg/day)	Iodine (µg/portion) (QCT: 150µg/day)	Manganese (mg/portion) (QCT: 1.4mg/day)	Selenium (µg/portion) (QCT: 40µg/day)	Zinc (mg/portion) (QCT: 9.4mg/day)
4	54	16	tr	tr	tr	tr	tr	tr
0	0	10	tr	tr	tr	tr	tr	tr
tr	10	6	0	0	tr	0	0	0
tr	24	4	tr	tr	0	0	0	tr
4	88	10	tr	tr	tr	tr	tr	tr
n	10	112	n	n	0	n	0	n
42	96	18	0.03	0.3	tr	0.1	tr	0.3
57	117	21	tr	tr	tr	tr	tr	tr
15	18	21	tr	tr	tr	tr	tr	tr
78	144	18	tr	0.6	tr	tr	tr	tr
9	216	21	0.12	1.5	n	tr	tr	tr
9	71	5	0.01	0.6	n	tr	tr	tr
16	138	9	0.08	1.1	n	0.1	tr	0.1
8	76	5	0.01	0.6	n	0.1	tr	tr
6	49	2	0.05	0.2	n	tr	tr	tr
6	29	5	0.02	0.2	n	tr	tr	tr
3	17	6	0.02	0.2	n	tr	tr	tr
10	tr	22	tr	tr	n	tr	tr	0.1
tr	tr	2	tr	tr	n	tr	tr	tr
tr	tr	3	tr	tr	n	tr	n	tr
tr	tr	tr	tr	tr	tr	tr	tr	tr

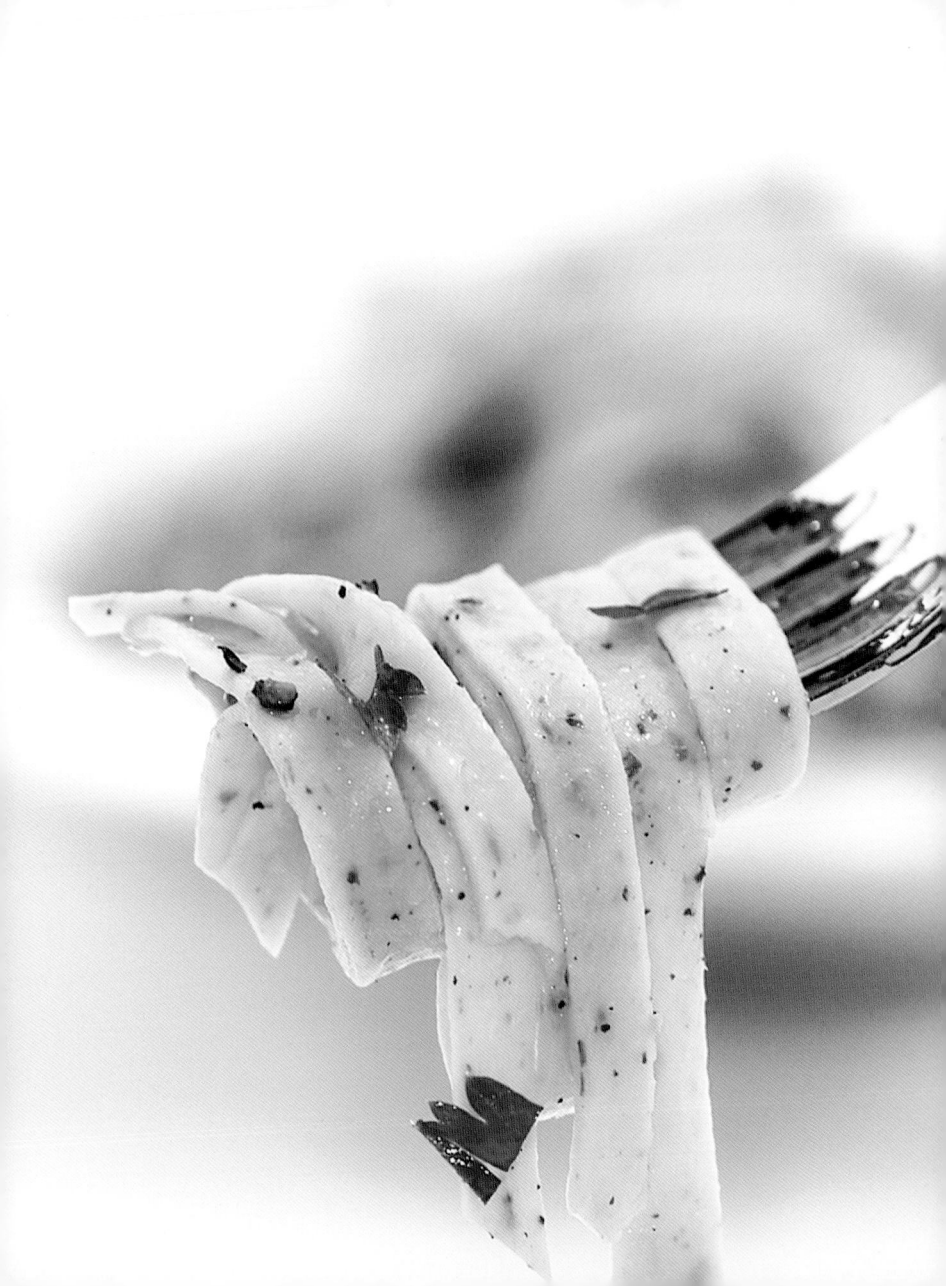

Part 4
DIETS

In this part we explore a range of strategies for achieving weight loss. We begin by looking at the importance of exercise and good nutrition for achieving sustained weight loss. This is followed by a review of a range of popular diets, including calorie-controlled diets, high-protein diets, low-fat diets and high-fat/low-carbohydrate diets. Next we are given some general principles for healthy slimming, and asked to consider the emotional triggers for over-eating. An "all-purpose" slimming plan provides a concrete example of how we can incorporate the principles of healthy dieting into our daily life. Then a 10-day detox and elimination diet takes us through the process of cutting out different foods, and then gradually reintroducing them. This enables us to find out which foods disagree with us.

Diets and dieting

The National Weight Control Registry (NWCR) – a national database of American individuals who have achieved successful weight loss – contains information on 2800 Americans over the age of 18 who have managed to maintain a 30 lb (13.5 kg) weight loss for a year or more. 55 per cent of those registered had participated in formal weight-loss programmes; 20 per cent had used low-calorie liquid diets; 4.3 per cent had used weight-loss medications; and 1.3 per cent had undergone gastric bypass surgery. Almost all had previously tried several weight-loss methods without success. Of those who were successful, 61 per cent followed a more rigorous diet than before, and 81 per cent exercised more. The average successful slimmer expended about 2800 kcal per week on exercise (about one hour a day). This evidence confirms that diet without exercise rarely produces lasting weight loss, and suggests that structured programmes make the process of dieting more effective.

As the majority of people wishing to lose weight also want to improve their long-term health, it is vital that slimming regimes incorporate the principles of healthy eating. Good nutrition is now accepted worldwide as the most powerful and cost-effective way of enhancing health and vitality, and of avoiding serious illness in the long term. A well-nourished body is better able to support and sustain weight loss than one fighting the effects of a poor diet.

Before looking at ways to make your slimming diet as healthy and effective as possible, here is a brief review of some popular weight-loss methods.

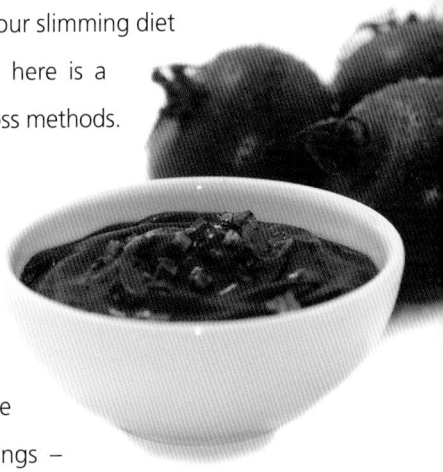

CALORIE-CONTROLLED DIETS

Calorie-controlled diets that restrict calorie intake to a daily maximum can certainly help us lose weight, but they also produce cravings – not only for more calories, but also for necessary nourishment. As it is not easy for us to distinguish between these two, we often find ourselves grabbing an illicit chocolate bar to provide some instant energy and a sense of relief and satisfaction.

Unfortunately, this satisfaction is often followed half an hour later by a headache and yet more cravings ... .

When calorie intake is restricted, the body changes its metabolism so that energy is provided from the burning up of fat stores. The change-over period lasts a few days and is usually accompanied by cravings, hunger, headaches and low energy levels. When we fast these symptoms are soon replaced by increased energy levels and heightened well-being. However, calorie-controlled diets tend to leave the body stuck in the change-over state, constantly craving food and feeling unwell.

HIGH-PROTEIN DIETS

In an attempt to avoid the negative effects of calorie control, some slimming diets advocate a very high protein intake. This is because the level of protein in the blood controls the brain's hunger-centre, so eating a protein-rich diet means you need to eat fewer calories to feel satisfied.

The downside is that a high-protein diet over a long period can cause quite severe health problems. This is because it may lack essential nutrients, phytochemicals and fibre and, more importantly, because the body has no way of storing the protein it doesn't need. Any excess is excreted and may cause kidney problems, so if you decide to follow a high-protein slimming regime, remember to drink plenty of water (at least two litres per day), and make sure that whatever carbohydrate you do eat comes from fresh plant foods that are high in fibre. If you intend to diet for an extended period, you should consult a qualified medical practitioner beforehand to ensure that you don't achieve weight loss at the expense of poor nutrition.

LOW-FAT DIETS

There is considerable debate about the role of excess dietary fat in the development of obesity, but it is clear from epidemiological studies that there is a worldwide association between high dietary fat intake and obesity. Laboratory studies on humans also show that individuals with access to high-fat foods will always eat these in preference to low-fat foods if given the choice, and that excess dietary fat is stored in the body with greater efficiency than excess dietary carbohydrate or protein. Diets designed to achieve weight loss by restricting fat intake have met with limited success, however. This may be because the body uses energy more efficiently when less is available.

HIGH-FAT/LOW-CARBOHYDRATE DIETS

As with high-protein diets, high-fat/low-carbohydrate diets can also reduce cravings because fats are calorie-dense, providing nine calories of energy per gram as opposed to only four calories per gram in carbohydrates and protein – which makes it possible to feel satisfied with smaller portions. Advocates of the "eat fat, grow slim" approach claim that fat is the least fattening of all foods because, when carbohydrate intake is restricted, eating more fat turns up the metabolic thermostat, mobilizing fat stores and burning up the food we eat more efficiently. Based on the idea that humans evolved as predators with a diet naturally high in fat and protein, high-fat enthusiasts claim that the degeneration of health (and the human condition) in modern times is due to the shift toward a diet based on "useless" carbohydrate fuel, such as cereals and grains.

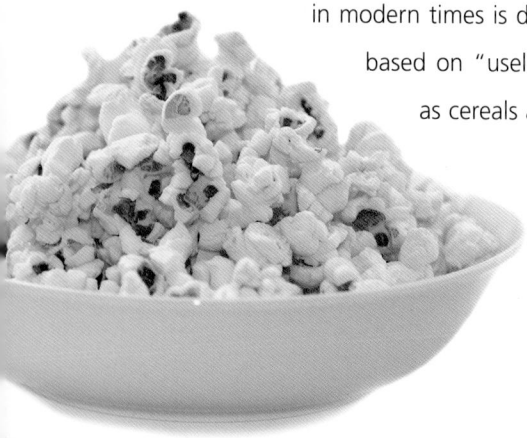

Although high-fat "stone age" diets have undoubtedly helped some people to lose weight, the balance of evidence suggests that most people would gain substantially more in health terms by increasing their intake of fresh fruits and vegetables, and moderating their intake of saturated fat.

GETTING THE MOST OUT OF YOUR SLIMMING DIET

Whatever type of slimming programme you choose, there are a number of nutritional and lifestyle guidelines that will help to ensure that your diet is as healthy and effective as possible:

- **Eat a balanced diet.** From a nutritional perspective, the best diet is high in complex carbohydrates (60–65 per cent), fibre and simple fruit sugars, and contains no refined sugar at all. It provides a moderate amount of protein (10–15 per cent), a controlled amount of unsaturated fat (20–30 per cent), and very little saturated fat.
- **Eat fresh fruits and vegetables.** The easiest way to improve your diet is to greatly increase your fruit and vegetable intake and cut out dairy products altogether. (There are plenty of non-dairy alternatives on the market including soya, rice, oat and almond milks, nut butters and pure vegetable margarines.)

- **Eat more fibre.** Fibre and complex carbohydrates are crucial for slimming because they are low in calories and yet give a feeling of fullness. They also improve fat and cholesterol metabolism, and aid digestion.
- **Eat proper meals.** To achieve weight loss it is better to eat proper meals than snacks. If you need to snack, eat natural wholefoods, such as wholemeal sugar-free biscuits, sugar-free cereal bars, carrot or celery sticks, bananas, papaya, apples and sugar-free dried fruits.
- **Pay attention to the quality of the fats you eat.** Cut down dairy and animal fat in your diet to a minimum and use olive oil (or other cold-pressed vegetable oils) for cooking. Avoid sources of saturated fats, such as lard, fatty meats, cream, cheese, butter and full-fat dairy products.
- **Drink plenty of water** – your body loses about 2.5 litres of water each day (depending on activity level and climate) in sweat, urine, faeces and breathing.
- **Stay off alcoholic beverages and sugary hot or cold drinks.** Exchange these for water, fruit juices, herb teas and chicory, dandelion or barley "coffees".
- **Start each meal with some fresh seasonal fruit.**

- **As far as possible, cut out all red and processed meats.** Steaks, burgers and sausages tend to be high in both total fat and saturated fat. Eat more seafood, poultry and pulses.
- **Beware of empty calories.** Avoid refined carbohydrates (such as added sugar, confectionery, biscuits and sweets), alcohol and processed snacks.
- **Read labels** – don't eat anything you don't agree with.
- **Eat papaya or grapefruit every day.** Both contain phytochemicals which complement the action of pancreatic digestive enzymes. Eating them can help you to decrease your calorie intake overall by making better use of the food you do eat.
- **Exchange black tea and coffee for green tea.** Green tea contains methylxanthines and antioxidants, which boost metabolism and immunity.
- **Add dandelion to your diet.** Dandelion root enhances fat digestion and is a traditional weight-loss remedy. The fresh root can be cooked like parsnip or stir-fried, and there are a number of roasted dandelion root "coffees" available in health stores. Dandelion leaves can be added to fresh salads.
- **Include potatoes in your diet.** Potatoes contain a protein that stimulates the release of a chemical called

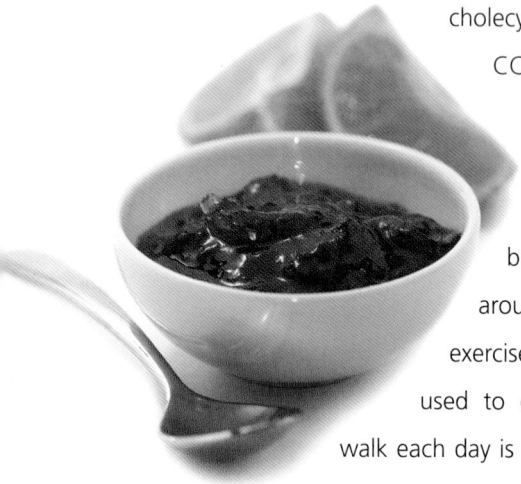

cholecystokinin (CCK). In the brain, CCK acts as a satiety factor, signalling to the body that it has had enough to eat.

- **Take daily exercise.** Fat-burning is most efficient at around 50 per cent of maximum exercise capacity, so if you are not used to exercising, a 20–30 minute walk each day is a good start. Try to establish a daily routine, but have one day off each week. Cycling, dancing, fitness training, swimming, running and stretching can all help to ensure that you make proper use of the food you eat. Obese individuals who achieve cardio-respiratory fitness have a lower mortality risk than sedentary people of normal weight, so even if weight loss is slow, exercise will do you good. Couch potatoes are jeopardizing their health, no matter how much they weigh.
- **Have breaks.** Rest is important for efficient digestion, so spend 15–30 minutes each day on relaxation or meditation. Taking short relaxation breaks during the day also decreases

the need for snacks to keep brain and body going.

- **Get fresh air whenever you can** and use it as an alternative to stimulants such as chocolate, tea and coffee to give you extra calorie-free energy.

DIET AND EMOTION

Eating satisfies the emotions as well as the stomach. The feelings of security and satisfaction that come from food can be traced back to infancy. Babies get very upset when they are hungry, and are easily calmed with food or by the sensation of eating (such as sucking a dummy or a finger).

All forms of stress, anxiety and fear eat up blood sugar and encourage us to reach for easy energy-fixes such as chocolate, cakes and snacks. Chronic stress is often soothed by thinking about, tasting, chewing and digesting food, and such patterns can be very resistant to change. Managing stress and paying attention to your emotional needs are therefore an integral part of successful weight loss. It is also important to understand the extent to which emotional factors influence your diet and eating habits, to ensure that you can maintain a healthy weight when the dieting is over.

Diet Plans

ALL PURPOSE SLIMMING DIET

When losing weight, it is important to eat foods that are low in calories, yet high in vitamins, minerals, trace elements, essential fatty acids and amino acids. It is also important to avoid stimulants (such as coffee, tea, chocolate and sugar). Dairy products, apart from live yogurt, are also best avoided. Follow the daily plan below to get started, and improvise using your own favourite quality calorie choices.

DAILY PLAN

ON RISING

- Drink a glass of water or unsweetened fruit juice.

BREAKFAST

- Drink a cup of herb tea, green tea, fruit juice or water.
- Eat half a grapefruit, followed by as much as you like of one of the following:
  - Fruit salad with added nuts and seeds.
  - Porridge with soya, rice or almond milk.
  - Low-fat live yogurt or soya yogurt with dried fruits (soaked overnight) and a few nuts and seeds sprinkled over the top.
  - Fruit followed by wholemeal bread with marmite or honey.

MID-MORNING

- Drink one glass of water or fruit juice, or a cup of herb tea.
- If you need a snack, eat some pieces of fruit, or some raw vegetable sticks

with oatcakes, crispbread or rice cakes topped with nut butter or low-fat spread.

LUNCH

- Eat at least two pieces of seasonal fruit; then a large plate of mixed salad with herbs (for example, thyme, parsley, watercress, marjoram), dressed with vinaigrette and accompanied by wholemeal bread, rice cakes, oatcakes or rye bread spread with houmous or nut butter.

MID-AFTERNOON

- Drink one glass of water or fruit juice or a cup of herb tea.
- If you feel hungry, eat some sticks of raw carrot, cucumber or celery, or some pieces of fruit, together with rice cakes, crackers or oatcakes.

EVENING MEAL

- Eat two pieces of seasonal fruit, followed by a portion of soup and a plate of food comprising one half green vegetables, one third root vegetables and/or grains, and one sixth fat/protein foods (see food groups below).

MID-EVENING

- Drink a cup of herb tea or a glass of water.

FRESH VEGETABLES: artichoke; asparagus; aubergine; bean sprouts; broccoli; brussels sprouts; cabbage; cauliflower; celery; courgette; cress; cucumber; curly kale; endive; fennel; green beans; leeks; lettuce; okra; onion; peas; peppers; pumpkin; spinach; spring greens; tomato.

ROOT VEGETABLES AND GRAINS: beetroot; bulgur wheat; carrot; celeriac; cereals; couscous; parsnip; potato; swede; sweetcorn; sweet potato; turnip; wholemeal bread; wholemeal pasta; wholegrain rice; wild rice.

FAT AND PROTEIN FOODS: avocado; dried beans; cheese; chick peas; crab; egg; fish; lean meat (including chicken and ham); lentils; mushrooms; nuts and seeds; olives; prawns; tempeh; tofu.

DETOX AND ELIMINATION

The best times to detox are spring and autumn. Carry it out at a time when you can take things easy. Don't be surprised or unnerved if you feel a little nauseous or headachy at first. When you detox, the waste products and toxins your body has stored in fat tissue are cleared away. The higher levels of toxins in your blood during this process can make you feel unwell. Don't lose heart – the symptoms will soon pass, leaving you feeling, lighter, more awake and more energetic than before. This diet involves gradually cutting certain drinks and foods out of your normal diet until you are drinking only water and grape juice. This is followed by the gradual reintroduction of different foods, one at a time, allowing you to see which ones agree with you and which do not.

10-DAY DETOX AND ELIMINATION

DAY 1

Eat normally but cut out tea, coffee, chocolate, alcohol, tobacco and fizzy drinks. Replace these with green tea, herb tea, fruit juice and plenty of water.

DAY 2

Cut out everything containing sugar. Replace these with fresh and dried fruit and nuts. Drink plenty of water

DAY 3

Cut out all meat and dairy products. If you are uncertain what to replace them with, try the following: for breakfast, the juice of one ruby-red grapefruit and muesli or porridge with dried fruits and nuts, served with soya, rice or almond milk; for lunch, mixed tofu and vegetable stir-fry, or mixed salad with rice; for an afternoon snack, fresh vegetable juice and fresh or dried fruit and nuts; for an aperitif, fresh vegetable juice; and for dinner, steamed vegetables and rice. Supplement these dishes with plenty of water between meals.

DAY 4

Cut out bread, rice, nuts and other grains. Eat plenty of fresh fruit and vegetables (raw or steamed). Drink plenty of unsweetened fruit juice and water.

DAY 5

Eat fruit only. Consume as much as you like (particularly grapes), whenever you like. Drink plenty of unsweetened fruit juice and water.

DAY 6

Drink only grape juice and plenty of water.

DAY 7

Eat fruit only. Consume as much as you like (particularly grapes), whenever you like. Drink plenty of unsweetened fruit juice and water.

DAY 8

Eat plenty of fresh fruit and vegetables (raw or steamed). Drink lots of unsweetened fruit juice and water.

DAY 9

Reintroduce grains, bread, rice and nuts. Eat lots of fresh fruit and vegetables, and drink plenty of unsweetened fruit juice and water.

DAY 10

Gently begin reintroducing your normal diet. Add one food type per day. Notice whether you experience any adverse reactions to particular items as you reintroduce them. If so, you may choose to cut these out of your diet altogether or at least limit your intake of them.

(Above all, after finishing your detox diet, don't rush out immediately for a big meal with wine and coffee – it could make you feel extremely unwell.)

Index

acrylamide 37
adenosine tri-phosphate 168
amino acids 38–40, 41
antioxidants 100, 178

basal metabolic rate (BMR) 24–27
beta-carotene 96, 98
body mass index (BMI) 28

cadmium 176
calcium 164–5
calorie-intake tables 29
calories 12–29
  see also quality calories
carbohydrate, fat and protein tables 49–93
carbohydrates 32–6
carotenoids 96–7
cholecystokinin (CCK) 233–4
cholesterol 36, 45, 46
copper 176

dieting
  and exercise 22, 26, 226, 234
  guidelines 231–5
diets
  all-purpose slimming 236–7
  calorie-controlled 227–8
  detox and elimination 238–9
  high-fat/low-carbohydrate 230–1
  high-protein 228–9
  low-fat 229
digestion
  carbohydrates 33–4
  and fibre 22
  protein 38

energy
  and calories 12–13, 24–7, 29
  energy needs 24–7
  and fats 12, 230
essential fatty acids (EFAs) 43–4, 46

fat cells 21
fats 42–8
fatty acids 42–4, 46–7
fibre 22, 32–3, 35–6, 41, 232
fluoride 176
free radicals 100–2

glucose 33

insulin 34, 39
iodine 177
iron 172–3

kilocalories 12

lipoproteins 45

magnesium 166–7
manganese 175–6
metabolism 12, 33, 175, 177, 228, 230
micronutrients 15–16
minerals 164–71
mineral and trace element tables 179–223
molybdenum 176
monounsaturated fatty acids 42–3, 46, 47

nutritional guidelines 231–4

obesity 20–3, 229
omega-3 fatty acids 44, 46
omega-6 fatty acids 43–4

phosphorus 167–9
phytochemicals 41, 233
polyunsaturated fatty acids 42, 43, 46, 47
potassium 169–70
protein 38–41
  and dieting 228–9
  needs 40–1

quality calories 14–15
  vs. empty calories 14
  counting 16, 17–18
quality-calorie targets (QCTs) 19–20

retinol 96–8

saturated fatty acids 42, 46, 47
selenium 178
sodium 169–70
sodium chloride 170–1
starch 33, 35

trace elements 172–8
trans fats 44, 47
tryptophan 109–10

vitamins, fat-soluble
  vitamin A 96–8
  vitamin D 98–100, 165, 168
  vitamin E 100–102
  vitamin K 102–3
vitamins, water-soluble
  biotin 118
  folate (folic acid) 116, 117
  vitamin B1 (thiamin) 106–7, 166
  vitamin B2 (riboflavin) 108
  vitamin B3 (niacin) 109–11
  vitamin B5 (pantothenate) 111–12
  vitamin B6 (pyridoxine) 113–15, 166, 174
  vitamin B12 (cobalamin) 114–17
  vitamin C 104–5
vitamin tables 119–63

zinc 173–4